Posterior and Plantar Heel Pain

Editor

ERIC A. BARP

CLINICS IN PODIATRIC MEDICINE AND SURGERY

www.podiatric.theclinics.com

Consulting Editor
THOMAS J. CHANG

April 2021 • Volume 38 • Number 2

ELSEVIER

1600 John F. Kennedy Boulevard • Suite 1800 • Philadelphia, Pennsylvania, 19103-2899

http://www.theclinics.com

CLINICS IN PODIATRIC MEDICINE AND SURGERY Volume 38, Number 2
April 2021 ISSN 0891-8422, ISBN-13: 978-0-323-79632-3

Editor: Lauren Boyle
Developmental Editor: Nicole Congleton

Clinics in Podiatric Medicine and Surgery (ISSN 0891-8422) is published quarterly by Elsevier Inc., 360 Park Avenue South, New York, NY 10010-1710. Months of issue are January, April, July, and October. Business and Editorial Offices: 1600 John F. Kennedy Blvd., Ste. 1800, Philadelphia, PA 19103-2899. Customer Service Office: 3251 Riverport Lane, Maryland Heights, MO 63043. Periodicals postage paid at New York, NY and additional mailing offices. Subscription prices are $310.00 per year for US individuals, $750.00 per year for US institutions, $100.00 per year for US students and residents, $382.00 per year for Canadian individuals, $776.00 for Canadian institutions, $462.00 for international individuals, $776.00 per year for international institutions, $100.00 per year for Canadian students/residents, and $220.00 per year for foreign students/residents. To receive student/resident rate, orders must be accompanied by name of affiliated institution, date of term, and the *signature* of program/residency coordinator on institution letterhead. Orders will be billed at individual rate until proof of status is received. Foreign air speed delivery is included in all *Clinics* subscription prices. All prices are subject to change without notice. POSTMASTER: Send address changes to *Clinics in Podiatric Medicine and Surgery*, Elsevier Health Sciences Division, Subscription Customer Service, 3251 Riverport Lane, Maryland Heights, MO 63043. **Customer Service: 1-800-654-2452 (US). From outside of the US, call 314-447-8871. Fax: 314-447-8029. E-mail: JournalsCustomerService-usa@elsevier.com (for print support); JournalsOnlineSupport-usa@elsevier.com (for online support).**

Reprints. For copies of 100 or more of articles in this publication, please contact the Commercial Reprints Department, Elsevier Inc., 360 Park Avenue South, New York, NY 10010-1710. Tel.: 212-633-3874; Fax: 212-633-3820; E-mail: reprints@elsevier.com.

Clinics in Podiatric Medicine and Surgery is covered in *MEDLINE/PubMed (Index Medicus)* and *EMBASE/Excerpta Medica*.

Contributors

CONSULTING EDITOR

THOMAS J. CHANG, DPM
Clinical Professor and Past Chairman, Department of Podiatric Surgery, California College of Podiatric Medicine, Faculty, The Podiatry Institute, Redwood Orthopedic Surgery Associates, Santa Rosa, California

EDITOR

ERIC A. BARP, DPM, FACFAS
Foot and Ankle Department, The Iowa Clinic, West Des Moines, Iowa; Residency Director, Podiatry, UnityPoint Health - Iowa Methodist Medical Center, Des Moines, Iowa

AUTHORS

ERIC A BARP, DPM, FACFAS
Foot and Ankle Department, The Iowa Clinic, West Des Moines, Iowa; Residency Director, Podiatry, UnityPoint Health - Iowa Methodist Medical Center, Des Moines, Iowa

ZACHARY J. BLIEK, DPM
The Iowa Clinic, UnityPoint Health - Iowa Methodist Medical Center, Des Moines, Iowa

DONALD BUDDECKE Jr, DPM, FACFAS
Private Practice, Foot and Ankle Surgery, Foot and Ankle Specialists, Omaha, Nebraska

ROBERT CAVALIERE, DPM
Second Year Resident, Highlands-Presbyterian, St. Luke's Podiatric Medicine and Surgery Residency Program, Denver, Colorado

JAMES M. COTTOM, DPM, FACFAS
Fellowship Director, Florida Orthopedic Foot and Ankle Center, Sarasota, Florida

WILLIAM T. DECARBO, DPM, FACFAS
Fellowship Trained Foot and Ankle Surgeon, Board Certified Foot and Ankle Surgeon, St. Clair Orthopedic Associates, Pittsburgh, Pennsylvania

SEAN T. GRAMBART, DPM, FACFAS
Assistant Professor and Assistant Dean of Academic Affairs, Des Moines University, College of Podiatric Medicine and Surgery, Attending Physician, UnityPoint Health - Iowa Methodist Medical Center, Des Moines, Iowa

NEPHI E.H. JONES, DPM
The Iowa Clinic, UnityPoint Health - Iowa Methodist Medical Center, Des Moines, Iowa

JAY LECHNER, BS
Podiatric Medical Student, Des Moines University, College of Podiatric Medicine and Surgery, Des Moines, Iowa

JEFFREY E. MCALISTER, DPM, FACFAS
Phoenix Foot and Ankle Institute, Scottsdale, Arizona

LAUREN MOLCHAN, DPM
Second Year Resident, Highlands-Presbyterian, St. Luke's Podiatric Medicine and Surgery Residency Program, Denver, Colorado

TRAVIS MOTLEY, DPM, MS, FACFAS
Professor and Program Director, Podiatric Surgical Residency, John Peter Smith Hospital, Acclaim Physician Group, Fort Worth, Texas

SCOTT C. NELSON, DPM, FACFAS
Department of Orthopedics, Catholic Health Initiatives (CHI Health), Omaha, Nebraska

ALAN NG, DPM, FACFAS
Advanced Orthopedic and Sports Medicine Specialists, Fellowship Director, Rocky Mountain Reconstructive Foot and Ankle Fellowship, Highlands-Presbyterian, St. Luke's Podiatric Medicine and Surgery Residency Program, Denver, Colorado

RYAN D. PRUSA, DPM, PGY2
The Iowa Clinic, UnityPoint Health - Iowa Methodist Medical Center, Des Moines, Iowa

RONALD G. RAY, DPM, FACFAS, WCC, PT
Benefis Foot and Ankle Clinic, Great Falls, Montana

ERIC R. REESE, DPM
The Iowa Clinic, UnityPoint Health - Iowa Methodist Medical Center, Des Moines, Iowa

CHARLES A. SISOVSKY, DPM, AACFAS
Fellow, Florida Orthopedic Foot and Ankle Center, Sarasota, Florida

ERIC W. TEMPLE, DPM
The Iowa Clinic, UnityPoint Health - Iowa Methodist Medical Center, Des Moines, Iowa

USMAN UROOJ, DPM, PGY-III
Department of Surgery-Podiatry, Chief Resident, Carl T. Hayden Medical Center, Phoenix, Arizona

JENNIFER WENTZ, BS
Podiatric Medical Student, Des Moines University, College of Podiatric Medicine and Surgery, Des Moines, Iowa

Contents

Tarsal tunnel syndrome is paresthesia and pain in the foot and ankle caused by entrapment and compression of the tibial nerve within the fibro-osseous tarsal tunnel beneath the flexor retinaculum. The most helpful diagnostic criteria are a positive Tinel sign at the ankle and objective sensory loss along the distribution of the tibial nerve. Treatment is designed to reduce the compression of the nerve, and surgical nerve release is indicated with failure of conservative options. It is important to identify the causative factor of the nerve compression and eliminate it to obtain excellent results.

Active individuals can experience exercise-induced pain along the medial, plantar central, and plantarmedial proximal arch. In many cases, these symptoms are consistent with conditions involving the plantar fascia, posterior tibial tendon, or entrapment of branches of the posterior tibial nerve. Unlike these other conditions, chronic exertional compartment syndrome (CECS) of the foot can be aggravated by interventions that impart any pressure or compression to the foot. Practitioners should have a high index of suspicion for CECS when classic treatments tend to aggravate patient's symptoms.

Calcification of the posterior portion of the calcaneus has numerous terms that refer to this pathology. Given the number of names, there can be confusion when discussing the different pathologies involving calcification at the insertion of the Achilles tendon at the calcaneus. Two of the diagnosis that can be confused with each other are Haglund's deformity and Achilles insertional calcific tendinosis. This article discusses how these 2 entities are differentiated clinically and how their surgical management is different.

Postoperative complications can be burdensome on both the patient and the surgeon. Attention in literature is often directed toward different forms of treatment and successful outcomes in surgery. The incentive of this article is to bring insight toward postoperative complications in rearfoot surgery, more specifically, the repair of the Achilles tendon with suture tape and suture anchors. This article directs attention to the recent reports on hypersensitivity reactions seen with the use of suture tape and nonabsorbable suture anchors and may encourage physicians to make patients aware of this potential complication when using these materials.

Many randomized controlled trials demonstrate the effectiveness of conservative treatment of plantar fasciitis. Patients with acute plantar fasciitis generally respond to treatment more rapidly and more predictably than patients with chronic plantar fasciitis. If conservative treatment fails, endoscopic plantar fasciotomy offers patients a more prompt return to activity compared with open procedures.

There is an ever-evolving debate about the best treatment option for Achilles tendon ruptures. There was a relative consensus that operative treatment yielded the best outcomes. Much of this is based on results in athletic populations. Conservative treatment was considered only for the elderly and those with very inactive lifestyles. There has been an evolution, however, with more surgeons utilizing an aggressive functional rehabilitation with conservative management. Surgical intervention still is the treatment of choice for elite-level athletes. The treatment of choice for patient populations other than elite athletes remains an individual choice between patient and physician.

Bone tumors of the foot are an uncommon finding. Most tumors are found incidentally on imaging and are benign. Care must be taken although due to the aggressive nature of malignant bone tumors that can occur in the calcaneus. Malignant lesions will more commonly present with symptoms of pain and swelling. Often misdiagnosed as soft tissue injuries, it is critical to be able to diagnose and treat these lesions early. Imaging plays an important role with plain films and advanced imaging. Surgical treatments can range from curettage with grafting to amputation for more aggressive lesions.

The treatment of Achilles tendinitis from conservative to minimally invasive to surgery gives patients a wide range of treatment options for this common pathology. The use and role of biologics to augment this treatment is emerging. The use of biologics may enhance the healing potential of the Achilles tendon when conservative treatment fails. There are a handful of biologics being investigated to obtain if improved outcomes can be maximized.

Alan Ng, Robert Cavaliere, and Lauren Molchan

Plantar fasciitis has been considered an acute inflammatory disorder. However, the local histologic findings represent a more chronic, degenerative state without inflammation. Patients may be stuck in a chronic state of cyclical inflammation leading to tissue degeneration, refractory symptoms, and disability. This idea process has influenced the treatment approach of some practitioners who have implemented the idea of regenerative medicine and use of biologic adjuvants in the treatment of plantar heel pain. Biologic therapies provide many different cellular components, growth factors, and proteins to restore normal tissue biology and are a useful adjunct in the treatment of recalcitrant plantar fasciitis.

James M. Cottom and Charles A. Sisovsky

 Video content accompanies this article at http://www.podiatric. theclinics.com/.

Achilles tendon ruptures are a common ailment and often missed in upwards of 25% of cases. Neglected Achilles injuries can be treated both conservatively and surgically. Physical therapy, bracing, and custom ankle-foot orthoses are some options to consider. Surgically, there are many options, depending on the quality of the existing tendon, size of the defect, and the surgeon's comfort with the technique. Those procedures include primary repair, V-Y tendon advancement, turndown flap, tendon transfers, and other allografts. These techniques have been shown to have good to excellent outcomes and typically return patients to activities without complaints.

Jeffrey E. McAlister and Usman Urooj

This article offers an overview of os trigonum syndrome, complications, operative techniques, and the authors' preferred protocol. Os trigonum is an ossicle like many other ossicles in the foot and ankle. Individuals who require repetitive plantarflexion of the ankle for activity may develop symptoms of an enlarged os trigonum. Usually, symptoms will be isolated to the posteriolateral aspect of the ankle. Because of the normal anatomic route of the flexor hallucis longus tendon, its range of motion may also elicit pain to the posterolateral ankle. Conservative, as well as surgical including both endoscopic and open excision, has been described.

CLINICS IN PODIATRIC MEDICINE AND SURGERY

FORTHCOMING ISSUES

July 2021
Cavus Foot Deformity
John Visser, *Editor*

RECENT ISSUES

January 2021
**OrthoplasticTechniques for Lower Extremity
Reconstruction - Part II**
Edgardo R. Rodriguez-Collazo and
Suhail Masadeh, *Editors*

October 2020
**OrthoplasticTechniques for Lower Extremity
Reconstruction - Part I**
Edgardo R. Rodriguez-Collazo and
Suhail Masadeh, *Editors*

SERIES OF RELATED INTEREST

*Orthopedic Clinics
Clinics in Sports Medicine
Foot and Ankle Clinics
Physical Medicine and Rehabilitation Clinics*

THE CLINICS ARE AVAILABLE ONLINE!
Access your subscription at:
www.theclinics.com

Foreword

Posterior and Plantar Heel Pain

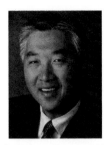

Thomas J. Chang, DPM
Consulting Editor

Heel pain is arguably the most common presentation in any foot and ankle clinic. Most clinics will likely see 10% to 20% of their new patients present with some form of heel pain, and most commonly plantar fasciitis. We are extremely capable of providing high-level treatment options for first-time patients, which include physical therapy techniques, oral and injectable anti-inflammatory medications, and supportive orthotic devices. Nonsurgical approaches have become the standard of care with early treatment and are 90% to 95% successful. But what about the other 5%?

In 1984, Dr Donald Baxter first described nerve entrapment syndrome as a possible cause of chronic heel pain. This heightened our awareness of neuritic contributions to heel pain and of other differential diagnoses besides mechanical. When standard treatment options for plantar fasciitis have failed, we need to be well versed in thinking outside the box.

I am grateful to Dr Eric Barp for taking a common and possibly redundant topic area and expanding this to current discussions on other causes of heel pain. His selection of respected authors offers an extensive breakdown of other causes, to include a variety of soft tissue and osseous pathologic conditions. Current concepts of orthobiologics are also presented in 2 different articles by Drs William DeCarbo and Alan Ng.

I hope you enjoy this issue. You will be introduced to new perspectives and likely impressed at how much we can learn in an area where we thought we already knew everything. I have been pleasantly surprised.

Thomas J. Chang, DPM
Redwood Orthopedic Surgery Associates
208 Concourse Boulevard
Santa Rosa, CA 95403, USA

E-mail address:
thomaschang14@comcast.net

Clin Podiatr Med Surg 38 (2021) ix
https://doi.org/10.1016/j.cpm.2021.01.002
0891-8422/21/© 2021 Published by Elsevier Inc.

podiatric.theclinics.com

Preface

Posterior and Plantar Heel Pain Pathologic Conditions

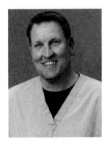

Eric A. Barp, DPM, FACFAS
Editor

It is a great honor to present this issue of *Clinics in Podiatric Medicine and Surgery* on "Posterior and Plantar Heel Pain." These are pathologic conditions that foot and ankle surgeons deal with daily and can be difficult to diagnose and manage. Foot and ankle surgeons must have deep knowledge on the differential diagnoses as well as treatment options for posterior and plantar heel pain. Often, these pathologic conditions present with similar signs and symptoms.

I deeply appreciate all of the authors that have contributed to this issue. I continually learn from each and every one of them whether it is via direct communication, watching them lecture, or bouncing cases off of one another. I thank all of them for taking the time out of their busy lives and practices to contribute. All are life-long learners and teachers, and I appreciate their dedication to the profession.

Please enjoy this issue. I believe the reader will find these articles beneficial to the practice of foot and ankle surgery.

Eric A. Barp, DPM, FACFAS
Foot and Ankle Department
The Iowa Clinic
5950 University Avenue
West Des Moines, IA 50266, USA

E-mail address:
ebarp@iowaclinic.com

Clin Podiatr Med Surg 38 (2021) xi
https://doi.org/10.1016/j.cpm.2021.01.001
0891-8422/21/© 2021 Published by Elsevier Inc.

podiatric.theclinics.com

Tarsal Tunnel Syndrome

Scott C. Nelson, DPM

KEYWORDS

- Tarsal tunnel syndrome • Tibial nerve • Nerve compression • Neuropathy

KEY POINTS

- Tarsal tunnel syndrome is characterized by paresthesia and pain in the plantar foot and medial ankle.
- Tinel sign, or paresthesia and pain when percussion of the tibial nerve, is a good clinical test for tarsal tunnel syndrome.
- It is important to identify the causation of the nerve compression, whether it be intrinsic or extrinsic to the foot.
- Advanced imaging and neurologic testing can aid in diagnosis of tarsal tunnel syndrome.

INTRODUCTION

The tarsal tunnel is located along the medial aspect of the ankle and foot and is considered a fibro-osseous space between the medial malleolus and the calcaneus. Several structures course through this anatomic space, including the tibial nerve, the posterior tibial artery and vein, the posterior tibial tendon, the flexor digitorum longus tendon, and the flexor hallucis longus tendon.[1] The tibial nerve passes between the FDL and FHL muscles before it bifurcates in the tarsal tunnel. The nerve branches at this level into the medial plantar nerve, lateral plantar nerve, and medial calcaneal nerve. In 5% of people, the bifurcation occurs before the tarsal tunnel. The medial and lateral plantar nerves proceed distally under the abductor hallucis muscle belly and its deep fascial covering. The soft tissue overlying these structures includes the flexor retinaculum or laciniate ligament and crural fascia proximally. Compression of the tibial nerve or one of its branches within the tarsal tunnel is the cause of the symptoms associated with the syndrome. The clinical symptoms typically are diffuse and poorly localized and often associated with paresthesia along the medial ankle and/or plantar foot (**Fig. 1**).

Department of Orthopedics, Catholic Health Initiatives (CHI Health), 16909 Lakeside Hills Court, Suite 208, Omaha, NE 68130, USA
E-mail address: Scn4dpm@gmail.com
Twitter: @docnelle (S.C.N.)

Clin Podiatr Med Surg 38 (2021) 131–141
https://doi.org/10.1016/j.cpm.2020.12.001
0891-8422/21/© 2021 Elsevier Inc. All rights reserved.

podiatric.theclinics.com

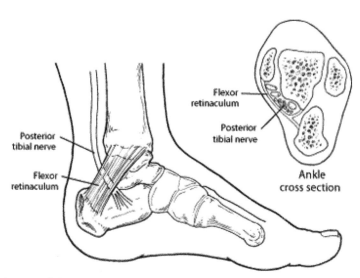

Fig. 1. Diagram of the anatomy of the tarsal tunnel. (*Reprinted with permission from* the American College of Foot and Ankle Surgeons. Available at: https://www.foothealthfacts. org/conditions/tarsal-tunnel-syndrome).

CAUSE

The cause of tarsal tunnel syndrome (TTS), by definition, is anything that can create a compression of the tibial nerve or its terminal branches.[2]

Often the cause is idiopathic with a possible insidious progression of symptoms. It may be helpful to evaluate the patient, and if TTS is suspected, then look to intrinsic or extrinsic causes of the compression.[3]

- Extrinsic causes:
  - Biomechanical abnormalities (valgus or varus rearfoot)
  - Anatomic abnormalities (tarsal coalition, middle facet)
  - Postoperative scar formation
  - Systemic diseases causing inflammatory arthropathies or tendinopathies
  - Generalized lower extremity edema
  - Trauma
  - Systemic inflammatory arthropathies
  - Diabetes
- Intrinsic causes:
  - Tendinopathy/tenosynovitis
  - Perineural tumor or scarring
  - Space-occupying lesions or masses (ganglion cyst, varicose veins, lipoma)

It is also important to consider proximal compression as a possible underlying factor, and the most likely source would be lumbar nerve root 4 and 5 (L4, L5) and sacral nerve root 1 (S1). Lower-back symptoms generally are implicated as a causative factor, especially in patients with bilateral complaints. Distal nerve problems, including Morton neuroma formation, can be present as well, mimicking TTS or a concomitant complaint. Plantar fasciitis or chronic plantar fasciosis is often a causative factor or is a concomitant complaint and will need to be evaluated thoroughly as well.

EVALUATION

Patient history is the most important step to begin with, as it can clue the foot and ankle surgeon in on crucial elements to make an accurate diagnosis. Often there may be several diagnoses to consider, and knowing how to differentiate is an importation skill to hone. With compression of the tibial nerve, there are a few physical examination findings that need to be evaluated, with first and foremost the biomechanical evaluation of the hindfoot and ankle. It is important to evaluate for rearfoot valgus or varus and whether this is reducible and flexible or rigid and nonreducible. Medial arch mobility should be evaluated to see if pes planus is present as well.

Percussion of the tibial nerve along the medial ankle to check for Tinel sign with distally directed paresthesia is a common finding.[2]

Much less common would be the proximal directed or Valleix sign. Dorsiflexion and eversion to re-create nerve compression is another physical test and is done with the ankle maximally dorsiflexed and everted with the metatarsophalangeal joints maximally dorsiflexed and held for 10 seconds to induce or exacerbate numbness or pain.[4] A modified Phalen test that is done by plantar flexion and inversion of the ankle can also be used to illicit paresthesia distally as well.

Weight-bearing radiographs of the foot and ankle should be obtained with close attention made to evaluate alignment issues, osseous growths, stress fractures, and/or middle facet coalition.

MRI is often invaluable in determining the cause. Tendon or joint synovitis, varicosities, ganglion cysts, nerve sheath tumors, and low-lying muscle belly can be visualized with this modality.

Electrodiagnostic studies, including electromyographic study and nerve conduction velocities (EMG/NCV), play a large role in determining the accurate diagnosis and can help to eliminate the presence of lumbosacral radiculopathy or peripheral neuropathy. Motor nerve conduction with distal motor latencies of 7.0 milliseconds or more and decreased amplitude of motor action potentials of abductor hallucis or abductor digiti minimi muscles are considered a positive finding but are much less reliable than sensory findings. The diagnosis of TTS can be confirmed by the nerve conduction study with prolonged terminal latency in 44% of cases and abnormal mixed and sensory nerve conduction in 86% and 94% of cases, respectively.[5] Prolonged sensory action potentials of more than 2.3 milliseconds would be a more likely finding. Electrodiagnostic testing is inaccurate, and a normal study does not exclude the diagnosis of TTS.[6,7]

CONSERVATIVE OPTIONS

It is important to evaluate the patient and pursue conservative options in an attempt to treat TTS conservatively. Performing conservative treatment helps to establish a good rapport with the patient and allows the treating foot and ankle surgeon to evaluate the patient for a period to see improvement and observe compliance.

The goal of conservative treatment is to decrease pain and inflammation and relieve the compressive forces on the tibial nerve. Identification of the causative factors would be helpful to direct treatment in an appropriate fashion. Modalities often considered would be oral nonsteroidal anti-inflammatory drugs (NSAIDs) or analgesic acetaminophen in many situations. Gabapentin, pregabalin, and tricyclic antidepressants are other oral options for pain relief, and topical medications, including NSAIDs and lidocaine, can be helpful. In the presence of ganglion formation, aspiration and corticosteroid injection can be beneficial but may require ultrasound guidance.

Physical modalities with therapy can be helpful especially if the causative factor is related to tenosynovitis. These modalities would include ultrasound, iontophoresis, phonophoresis, and electrical stimulation. Strengthening exercises and calf muscle stretching can aid in tissue mobility and nerve mobility/gliding. If mechanical issues are in play, then kinesiology taping or custom-molded orthotics can help to reduce medial tension on the foot and ankle. A CAM (controlled, ankle, motion) boot may be required to reduce tissue stress and relieve nerve traction. If conservative measures have failed to relieve the symptoms, the patient would be a candidate for surgical release.

SURGICAL
Case 1

Nerve sheath tumor

A 69-year-old man presented with left foot and ankle pain with abnormal sensations into the plantar foot and medial forefoot for 1-year duration. He had tried accommodative orthotics and gabapentin and previous steroid injection without success. His physical examination showed no biomechanical abnormalities with normal pulses with a positive Tinel sign along the medial ankle.

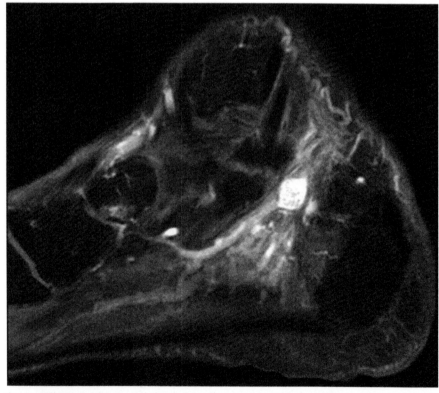

Fig. 2. MRI T2-weighted axial image of the presence of a nerve sheath tumor within the tibial nerve causing TTS.

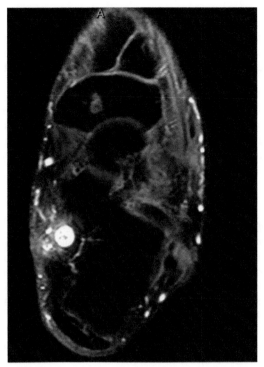

Fig. 3. MRI T2-weighted sagittal view of the tibial nerve sheath tumor.

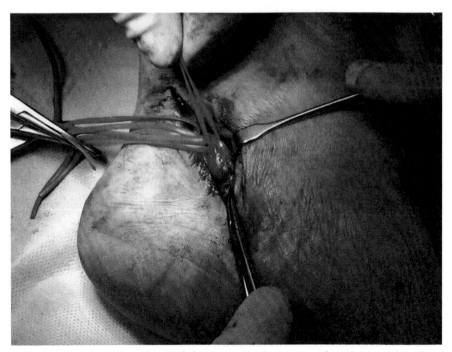

Fig. 4. Intraoperative photograph of the nerve sheath tumor, and corticosteroid residue is visible around the nerve from the previous injection.

MRI findings showed a cysticlike mass within the medial ankle and favored a nerve sheath tumor (schwannoma). The author thought with this finding there was no need to proceed with an EMG/NCV, and the recommendation was made for removal of the nerve tumor.

The nerve sheath tumor was completely excised, and in doing so, the nerve fascicles had to be individually separated under ×3.5 loops magnification to identify the individual fascicle that was involved. Once this was completed, the tumor was sectioned and sent to the pathology department for identification of schwannoma.

Postoperatively, the patient had return to full function and no apparent sensory abnormalities upon discharge (**Figs. 2–5**).

Case 2

Tarsal tunnel syndrome chronic plantar fasciosis

A 60-year-old woman presented with clinical left heel pain that extended into her arch of 18 months' duration. She had treatment of plantar fasciitis with corticosteroid injections, arch supports, physical therapy, and oral NSAIDs without long-term success. She had progression of her symptoms and developed a positive Tinel sign clinically. TTS was suspected, and the patient had an MRI and EMG/NCV performed to determine a surgical solution.

The MRI demonstrated thickened plantar fascial tissue (>8 mm) with inflammation. There was changes on her NCVs to indicate tibial nerve compression with sensory nerve involvement (**Figs. 6–9**).

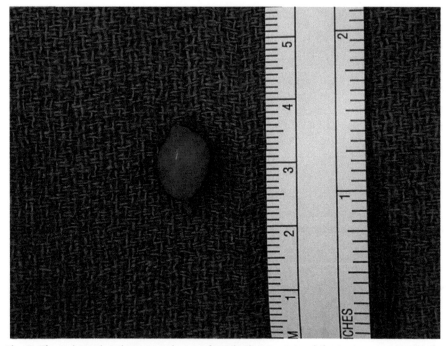

Fig. 5. The enlarged and separated nerve fascicle that contained the tumor was sent to the pathology department for identification of schwannoma.

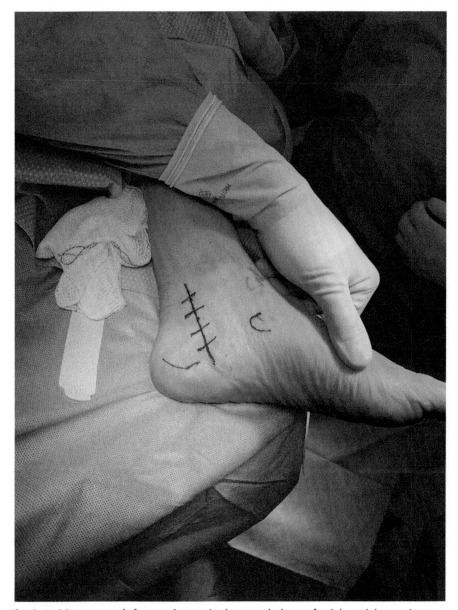

Fig. 6. Incision approach for tarsal tunnel release and plantar fascial partial resection.

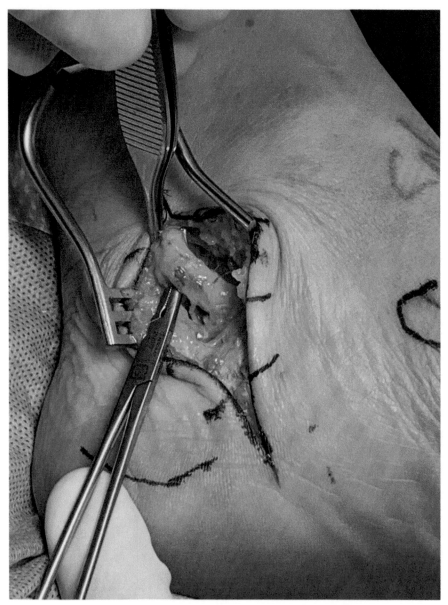

Fig. 7. Identification of the tibial nerve as it courses beneath the abductor hallucis muscle fascia.

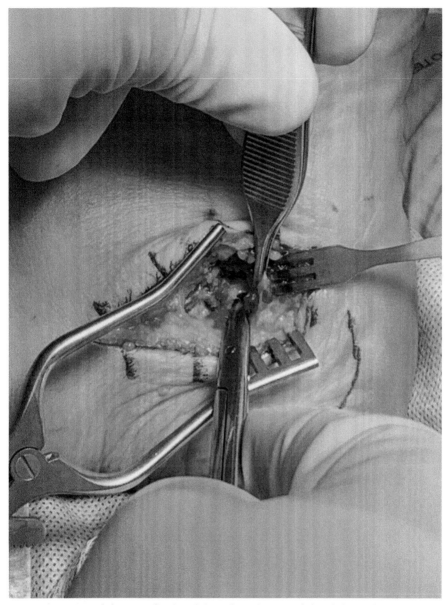

Fig. 8. Sectioning of the superficial and deep fascial tissue of the abductor hallucis muscle for completion of the tarsal tunnel release.

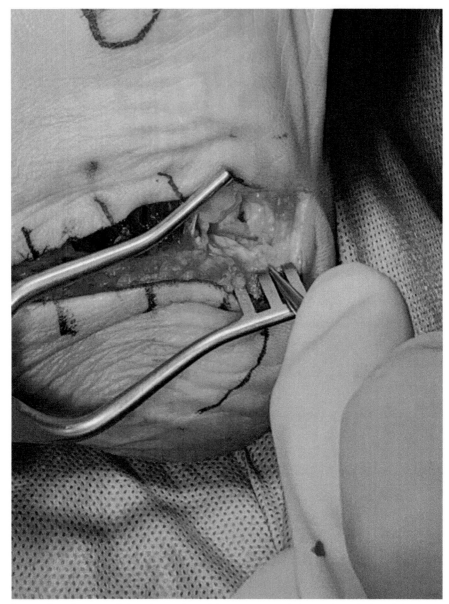

Fig. 9. Identification of the plantar fascial for resection of the thickened medial band.

SUMMARY

TTS is a clinical condition that is often difficult to identify and treat in a timely manner. It is important to consider this as a potential source of pain, and a thorough clinical examination should be done if this is suspected. The cause of nerve compression will often require advanced imaging and a thorough biomechanical examination of the foot and ankle. If conservative measures fail, a surgical release of the tibial nerve and its terminal branches can help in relieving the pain and parasthesia associated with compression.

DISCLOSURE

The authors have nothing to disclose.

REFERENCES

1. Cimino WR. Tarsal tunnel syndrome: review of the literature. Foot Ankle 1990;11(1): 47–52.
2. McSweeney SC, Cichero M. Tarsal tunnel syndrome-a narrative literature review. Foot 2015;25:244–50.
3. Komagamine J. Bilateral tarsal tunnel syndrome. Am J Med 2018;131(7):319.
4. Kinoshita M, Okuda R, Morikawa J, et al. The dorsiflexion-eversion test for diagnosis of tarsal tunnel syndrome. J Bone Joint Surg AM 2001;83-A(12):1835–9.
5. Oh SJ, Meyer. RD entrapment neuropathies of the tibial nerve. Neurol Clin 1993; 17(3):593–615.
6. Mann RA, Man RA, Coughlin MJ. Disease of the nerve. Surg foot Ankle 1999;2: 512–6. St Louis: Mosby.
7. Oh SJ. Tarsal tunnel syndrome encyclopedia of the neurological sciences. Waltham (MA): Academic Press/Elsevier; 2014. p. 391–3.

Chronic Exertional Compartment Syndrome of the Foot

Ronald G. Ray, DPM, WCC, PT

KEYWORDS

- Chronic compartment syndrome • Exertional compartment syndrome • Foot
- Foot compartment

KEY POINTS

- Chronic exertional compartment syndrome (CECS) of the foot most commonly involves the medial compartment followed by the superficial central compartment.
- Vascular inflow abnormalities can closely mimic symptoms commonly seen with CECS of the foot.
- It is prudent to conduct a thorough evaluation of a patient's vascular system to rule out pathology.
- Conservative measures are typically ineffective or aggravate a patient's condition, including the use of arch taping techniques, orthotic therapy, compression therapy, or lower extremity strengthening.
- Advanced imaging to evaluate structures within the lower leg, ankle, and foot is typically negative.
- Surgical release of the medial compartment (and possibly the superficial central compartment) can reduce or eliminate a patient's symptoms.

INTRODUCTION

Active patients, especially athletes, can present with exercise-induced pain in the plantarmedial proximal, plantarmedial central, and/or medial central arch. Patients presenting with symptoms in one or more of these regions may have a variety of conditions, including the following:

1. Plantar fasciitis
2. Lower tarsal tunnel/porta pedis entrapment of the lateral plantar nerve and/or its branches
3. Posterior tibial tendon insertional tendinosis
4. Sprain of the talonavicular joint or other medial column articulations
5. Anterior tibial tendon insertional tendinosis

Benefis Foot and Ankle Clinic, 1301 11th Avenue South, Suite 6, Great Falls, MT 59405, USA
E-mail address: drronray61@gmail.com

Clin Podiatr Med Surg 38 (2021) 143–164
https://doi.org/10.1016/j.cpm.2020.12.002
0891-8422/21/© 2020 Elsevier Inc. All rights reserved.

podiatric.theclinics.com

Another condition that needs to be considered in the differential diagnosis of medial arch pain is chronic exertional compartment syndrome (CECS) of the medial and superficial central compartments of the foot.

Exercise-induced compartment pain (not related to acute injury) has a lengthy history in the medical literature. It may have been first described in 1912 by Dr. Edward Wilson, the medical officer on Captain R.F. Scott's expedition to the South Pole. Dr. Wilson experienced pain and swelling in the anterior compartment of his leg with prolonged walking.[1] Horn[2] described a case of ischemic muscle necrosis that was presented in 1943 by Vogt to the Oregon State Medical Society. In 1944, 2 more cases were reported effecting an anterior/lateral compartment and an isolated anterior compartment.[2] In 1956, Mavor[3] described chronic recurrent exertional compartment syndrome of the anterior compartment in a football player who experienced bilateral recurrent exertional leg pain with muscle herniation and anterior ankle numbness. Since Mavor's[3] paper in 1965, there have been numerous case presentations and investigations on CECS of the leg.

CECS of the foot does not have a lengthy legacy compared with CECS of the leg. The concept of CECS of the foot was first mentioned in 1990 by Bouche.[4] Since its brief description in 1990, there have only been 13 cases (17 patients) in the literature.[5–12]

ETIOLOGY OF CHRONIC EXERTIONAL COMPARTMENT SYNDROME

Although speculative, theories concerning the pathophysiology of compartment syndrome propose that an increase in intracompartmental pressure results in compromised tissue perfusion. The role of ischemia in compartment syndrome has been challenged by MRI studies that indicate increased fluid within a compartment (not ischemia) may cause CECS.[13] Increased tissue pressure may result from limited or decreased compartment volume (ie, tight, noncompliant fascia), increased compartment content (ie, muscle swelling and hypertrophy), and externally applied pressure (ie, constricting hosiery, shoes, casts). Noncompliant fascia has been challenged as a contributor to CECS pathogenesis.[14]

Several theories attempt to explain compromised tissue perfusion in compartment syndrome. These include arterial spasm, critical closure, capillary occlusion, and arteriovenous gradient theories. Eaton and Green[15] speculated that increased compartment pressure produces local arterial spasm by a nonsympathetically mediated antidromic reflex leading to muscle ischemia. Burton[16] and Ashton[17] thought that if tissue pressure rises significantly or if arteriolar perfusion pressure drops, the gradient may decrease below critical closing pressure required for vessel patency. Ashton[17,18] and Hargens and colleagues[19] proposed the microvascular occlusion theory, in which tissue pressure rises above intracapillary pressure causing passive collapse of the soft-walled capillaries. The arteriovenous gradient theory described by Matsen and colleagues[20] includes increased tissue pressure resulting in increased local venous pressure, reduced local arteriovenous gradient, reduced local blood flow and oxygenation, and compromised tissue function/viability. Despite compromised tissue perfusion, peripheral pulses and digital circulation may remain intact. These theories are likely complementary, and each should be considered.

THE LAYERS AND COMPARTMENTS OF THE FOOT

The soft tissue structures of the plantar foot may be organized into several layers or grouped into various compartments. Knowledge of the anatomic layers provides spatial orientation from superficial to deep, as well as from side to side. The intermuscular septae in conjunction with the deep fascia divide the plantar soft tissues into discrete regions or compartments.

The plantar soft tissues can be divided into 4 layers from superficial to deep.[21–23] The first layer consists of the abductor hallucis, flexor digitorum brevis, and abductor digiti minimi. The main branches of the medial plantar artery and nerve pass between the abductor hallucis and flexor digitorum brevis before splitting into distal branches. The second layer consists of the quadratus plantae, 4 lumbricals, flexor hallucis longus tendon, and flexor digitorum longus tendon. Coursing from medial to lateral between the first and second layers are the lateral plantar artery and nerve. The third layer consists of the flexor hallucis brevis, adductor hallucis, and flexor digiti minimi. The fourth layer consists of 3 plantar and 4 dorsal interossei, the peroneus longus tendon and the posterior tibialis tendon.[21–23]

The foot also can be divided into compartments.[24–30] Most investigators agree there are 3 main plantar compartments and a less well defined dorsal compartment. The plantar compartments are the medial, central, and lateral. The structure of these compartments is varied among investigators. Beginning with the medial compartment, the superficial and portions of the medial boundary are made up of the medial segment of the plantar aponeurosis.[30] The medial intermuscular septum marks the lateral-most extent of the medial compartment, which originates from the central component of the plantar aponeurosis. Observations by Martin[31] reveal that the medial intermuscular septum divides into proximal, middle, and distal bands. Each band has a medial and lateral division. Although the medial intermuscular septum is a formidable structure, with no apparent direct communication occurring between the medial and central compartments,[31] injection studies as well as patterns of infection have shown passage of material from the medial into the central compartment.[25,32] The floor of the medial compartment is made up of the navicular, medial cuneiform, and first metatarsal. Structures within the medial compartment include abductor hallucis, flexor hallucis brevis, medial plantar nerve, and branches of the medial plantar artery. In contrast, Kamel and Sakla[33] found the abductor hallucis to be the sole occupant within the medial compartment, whereas the flexor hallucis brevis and oblique head of the adductor hallucis existed within the central compartment. A potential space exists between the abductor hallucis and the flexor hallucis brevis, providing a potential pathway for infection.[24]

The central compartment is bordered medially and laterally by the intermuscular septae. The superficial boundary is the central component of the plantar aponeurosis. Superiorly, the compartment is limited by the interossei and metatarsals 2, 3, and 4. The central compartment has been divided into various subcompartments.[24–33] There is disagreement among investigators regarding the number, extent, and make-up of these subcompartments.

Generally, 3 main subcompartments have been identified: superficial, middle or intermediate, and deep. The superficial subcompartment contains the flexor digitorum brevis and distal portions of the flexor digitorum longus tendons.[29,31,33] The proximal extent of this compartment is the medial tuberosity of the calcaneus and distally extends to the confluence of the flexor tendons and lumbricals. The intermediate subcompartment houses the quadratus plantae, proximal segments of the flexor digitorum longus and lumbrical muscles.[30] Manoli and Weber[29] identified the quadratus plantae as being housed within its own unique compartment ("Calcaneal Compartment") based on injection studies. They presented 3 cases of calcaneal fractures that subsequently developed lesser digital clawing due to ischemic contracture of the quadratus plantae. Sarrafian[30] placed the interossei along with the adductor hallucis (both oblique and transverse components) within the deep subcompartment of the central compartment. Other investigators have described the adductor hallucis as being encased within its own unique compartment, separate from the interossei muscles.[29,34]

In contrast, Kamel and Sakla[33] found a horizontal "Y"-shaped septum that defined the 3 subcompartments within the central compartment. According to their dissections, the intermediate subcompartment contained the adductor hallucis, flexor hallucis brevis, and flexor hallucis longus tendon. The deep subcompartment contained only the dorsal and plantar interossei. In contrast to several other investigators, Kamel and Sakla[33] placed the flexor digitorum brevis, quadratus plantae and the lumbricales in a separate compartment.

Although Kamel and Sakla[33] placed all the interossei within the deep subcompartment of the central compartment, other investigators[26–30] have described 4 unique compartments for the interossei. Three vertical septae extend inferiorly from the central 3 metatarsals to the deep fascia enclosing the adductor compartment (which is contained within its own compartment). Evidence for the interossei being within their own compartments is seen clinically following crush injuries to the foot where high intracompartmental pressures necessitate surgical decompression of the individual compartments.[26–28]

Grodinsky[24] also identified 4 potential spaces within the central compartment. The first space (M1) is between the plantar aponeurosis and the flexor digitorum brevis. It can have thin septae dividing it into 4 separate compartments from proximal to distal. These septae can be easily disrupted allowing free communication through the space. M2 is triangular space between the flexor digitorum brevis and quadratus plantae. Within its potential space, the lateral plantar artery and nerve cross. M3 is also a triangular potential space anterior and deep to M2. M3 is beneath the quadratus plantae, yet superficial to the adductor hallucis and its fascia. The floor of M3 is made up of the tarsal bones and accompanying ligaments. M4 lies anterior to M3 and deep to the adductor hallucis, but superficial to the fascia, forming the floor of the interossei compartments. Branches from the lateral plantar artery and nerve traverse through M4.

The lateral and superficial boundaries of the lateral compartment are marked by the plantar aponeurosis; medially, it is limited by the lateral intermuscular septum.[30] The abductor digiti minimi and flexor digiti minimi are found within this compartment. The floor is made of the plantar aspect of the fifth metatarsal, cuboid, and calcaneus. The lateral plantar neurovascular bundle enters the compartment proximally, travels along the lateral aspect of the lateral intermuscular septum, then leaves the compartment distally to reenter the central compartment. Grodinsky[24] identified a potential space within the lateral compartment between the flexor digiti minimi and abductor digiti minimi.

CLINICAL EXAMINATION
Patient History

Patients with CECS of the foot experience intermittent pain along the medial and plantar medial aspects of the arch, primarily in the middle and proximal one-third with activity. The arch becomes increasingly tight, which can progress into intense cramping. There is frequently localized swelling and excessive skin tension through the arch with or without redness. Complaints of tingling or numbness are inconsistent. Most patients tolerate a unique duration and intensity of exercise before symptoms stop activity. Symptoms can be brought on more rapidly with greater intensity if the foot is firmly enclosed by tape, compression stockings, or shoegear.

Physical Examination

An examination at rest reveals palpable lower extremity pulses and intact neurologic signs, including symmetric sensory and motor tests. In a number of cases, the abductor hallucis can be hypertrophied, especially in the proximal one-third of the arch. Some individuals will have a vertical zone of tenderness over the abductor hallucis consistent with the course of the lateral plantar and infracalcaneal nerves. There can also be a horizontal zone (angling downward from proximal to distal) of tenderness along the upper one-quarter of the abductor hallucis at the junction of the proximal and middle one-third of the arch. This zone of tenderness is consistent with the course of the medial plantar nerve. Superficial/medial and inferior fascial restrictions around the abductor hallucis associated with CECS can transfer pressure onto the branches of the posterior tibial nerve deep to the muscle. Evaluation immediately after activity continues to reveal an intact neurovascular system. The abductor hallucis can be diffusely tender, enlarged, and firm/tense. Greater tenderness may be appreciated when palpating the abductor hallucis overlying the branches of the posterior tibial nerve.

DIFFERENTIAL DIAGNOSIS

Clinical entities, whose presentation may be similar to CECS of the foot, can be organized into disease states affecting the vascular, neurologic, and musculoskeletal systems (**Table 1**). Vascular embarrassment to the limb can be caused by intrinsic disease of the vessel wall, embolic states, or extrinsic compressive syndromes. The most common form of intrinsic vessel disease is atherosclerosis, which involves invasion of the intima's endothelium by lipids and subsequently macrophages. This can generate a primary lesion in the vessel wall.[35] Over time, the lesion can fibrose, necrose, and ulcerate into the lumen, generating a localized thrombus. The vicious cycle results in calcification of the vessel wall and reduced elasticity. Vessel damage is most common near bifurcations (aortoiliac, femoropopliteal, and tibioperoneal).

Table 1
Differential diagnosis of chronic exertional compartment syndrome (CECS)

Vascular	Neurologic	Musculoskeletal
Adductor outlet	First branch, lateral	Abductor hallucis muscle
CECS of the foot	plantar nerve entrapment	herniation
Chronic arterial occlusive	Medial calcaneal nerve	Abductor hallucis muscle/
disease disorders	entrapment	tendon injury
(arteriosclerosis obliterans,	Medial plantar nerve	Accessory/Hypertrophic
aortoiliac arterial occlusive	entrapment	abductor hallucis muscle
disease, thromboangiitis	Proximal nerve disorders	Accessory navicular/Os
obliterans)	(eg, tibial nerve	navicularis
Popliteal adventitial cystic	entrapment, lumbar	Deep flexor tendinopathy
disease	radiculopathy, sciatica,	(ie, flexor hallucis longus
Popliteal artery entrapment	spinal stenosis)	tenosynovitis)
syndrome	Tarsal tunnel syndrome	Plantar fasciitis/Heel spur
	(proximal or distal tunnel)	syndrome
		Posterior tibial tendon
		insertional tendinosis
		Posterior tibial tendon
		dysfunction
		Postural pain (foot fatigue -
		from biomechanical
		etiology)
		Neoplasms (soft tissue
		or bone)
		Stress fracture
		(eg, calcaneus, navicular)

Tibioperoneal atherosclerosis can generate claudication symptoms within the superficial and deep posterior compartments of the leg, as well as the arch of the foot.

Entrapment syndromes of the femoral or popliteal artery involve impingement or compression of the vessel wall due to the vessel coursing through the local anatomy in an unusual or compromising fashion.[36–38] Popliteal artery entrapment was first described in 1965 by Love and Whelan.[39] Symptoms of claudication in the calf and/or foot along with coolness or blanching within the foot in primarily healthy young men (<30 years) should make one suspicious of popliteal artery entrapment.[36,37] Several classification systems categorize variations of the popliteal artery through the popliteal fossa. No classification is complete in its description of the artery's course.[40–42] The different categories take into account the following variations in popliteal fossa anatomy:

1. Aberrant course of the popliteal artery around the medial head of the gastrocnemius.
2. Lateral origin of the medial head of the gastrocnemius interfering with a normal coursing popliteal artery.
3. Accessory slips of the medial head of the gastrocnemius arising from a lateral location.
4. Variations in the popliteus origin or fibrous bands coursing through the popliteal fossa impinging the artery.[38–42]

In addition, popliteal aneurysms have been found in conjunction with popliteal artery entrapment, which represents a greater threat to the limb.[38] Imaging modalities to assist in the evaluation of the location and extent of this process have included ultrasonography, angiography, computed tomography (CT) scan, and MRI.

The popliteal artery also can receive compression from an adventitial mucin-containing cyst within the arterial wall, but not directly involving the media or intima.[43] This was first described by Ejurp and Hierton in 1954.[44] There are different theories as to the cause of cystic adventitial arterial degeneration, the most popular being that cysts develop from para articular ganglia arising from rests of scleroblastema.[45] Adventitial cysts have a lining of synovialike cells with the capacity to generate muciform fluid rich in hyaluronic acid.[43] Pedicles can exist between the knee joint and the cyst, contributing to fluctuations of fluid volume within the cyst, resulting in intermittent ischemia.[43,46] Pedicle formation may explain the longer recovery of claudication symptoms in patients with adventitial cystic disease. During activity, high fluid pressures generate within the knee joint (1000 mm Hg), forcing fluid into the adventitial cyst, increasing arterial pressure. Resorption of cyst fluid into the knee joint is delayed until fluid pressures within the knee normalize.[47]

Adventitial cystic disease of the popliteal artery occurs primarily in young nonsmoking adults who experience abrupt or gradual onset of claudication symptoms in the lower extremity. Physical examination reveals diminished to absent popliteal and pedal pulses depending on the degree of arterial compression or if thrombosis exists.[48] Murmurs or bruits may be auscultated over the popliteal fossa secondary to arterial narrowing. Flexion of the knee may exaggerate popliteal artery compression with a resultant loss of pedal pulses, along with pallor and coldness of the foot (Ishikawa sign).[49] Arterial Doppler pressures at rest are usually normal but reduce to abnormal levels during exercise. Angiography demonstrates normal arterial vasculature above and below the stenosed portion of the popliteal artery along with an absence of collateral flow. It is not uncommon for the popliteal artery to be displaced medially or laterally, depending on cyst dimensions.[47] Minor cyst involvement may be better demonstrated if the run-off is performed with the knee flexed to facilitate arterial compression. Extent of cyst involvement can also be evaluated effectively with ultra-sonography, CT scan, or MRI.[46,47]

Arterial compression can also occur more proximally within the boundaries of the adductor canal.[50,51] The adductor canal (Hunter canal) is a fascial tunnel through which the femoral artery/vein and saphenous nerve travel to access the popliteal fossa. The vastus medialis provides the anterior and lateral boundaries. The floor of the tunnel is made up of the adductor longus and adductor magnus. The roof of the tunnel consists of a strong layer of fascia above which the sartorius lies.[52] Adductor canal outlet syndrome most commonly involves compression of either the femoral artery/vein or saphenous nerve by hypertrophic tendinous bands extending between the adductor magnus and vastus medialis. Long-standing arterial compression can cause intrinsic injury resulting in intimal tears and subsequent arterial thrombosis. Patients will complain of intermittent claudication in the calf and foot, and paresthesias within the midfoot or forefoot in association with activity due to saphenous nerve entrapment. Symptoms may come on gradually and present intermittently in association with activity or present more acutely with intimal injury. On physical examination, the clinician may find diminished or absent popliteal or pedal pulses. Arterial Doppler examination may demonstrate reduced ankle pressure along with a profound drop after exercise. Increasing pallor and coolness may be appreciated at or below the knee, even after minimal activity.[50,51] Arteriograms are very effective at demonstrating the level and extent of occlusion present within the superficial femoral artery.

Peripheral nerve entrapment syndromes present features similar to CECS of the foot. Superficial peroneal nerve entrapment or tarsal tunnel syndrome can present in isolation or in combination with CECS of the foot. Superficial peroneal nerve entrapment was first described in 1945 by Henry[53] and was called "mononeuralgia in the superficial peroneal nerve." Adkison and colleagues[54] reviewed the variations in the course of the superficial peroneal nerve in 85 legs (44 cadavers) and found the nerve within the lateral compartment of the leg in 73% of specimens. Fourteen percent of the specimens had nerves exiting the anterior compartment fascia. Ten percent had branches exiting both the anterior and lateral compartments. Four percent of the nerves coursed superficial to the peroneus longus. Ultimately, the superficial peroneal nerve courses through a fascial tunnel before exiting through an opening in the deep fascia of the leg. Normally, the peroneal tunnel is less than 3 cm in length.[55] In some individuals, the nerve must navigate through a much longer tunnel, which may result in chronic nerve impingement. The peroneal tunnel may also become fibrotic around the nerve.[56] Excessive compression and tractioning on the superficial peroneal nerve may occur due to muscle herniation through an opening in the deep fascia.[56] Peroneal nerve irritation compounds when a patient presents with both muscle herniation through the deep fascial opening and a CECS of the anterior compartment.[57] The common peroneal nerve or one of its branches can also become entrapped as the nerve courses around the fibular neck, deep to the origin of the peroneus longus.[58]

Superficial peroneal nerve entrapment frequently elicits paresthesias and dysesthesias extending down the anterolateral aspect of the leg into the dorsal foot.[59] Exertion exacerbates symptoms including muscle weakness.[55,58,60] Onset of symptoms follows direct or indirect trauma in 25% of cases.[53,61,62] Rearfoot inversion sprains are a common cause of superficial peroneal nerve injury due to tractioning.[55,63] The onset of symptoms is more likely to occur following an inversion injury if the patient also possesses anatomic anomalies of the superficial peroneal nerve (ie, long peroneal tunnel, muscle herniation through the deep fascial opening, and/or exertional compartment syndrome). Several provocation tests have been described by Styf and Morberg[64] as a means of reproducing symptoms. The first maneuver involves having the patient actively dorsiflex the ankle joint while the clinician presses on the anterior intermuscular septum. The second and third maneuvers involve plantar flexing and inverting the foot with and without percussion over the nerve, respectively.[64] Multiple investigators describe the presence of a positive Tinel sign along the course of the superficial peroneal nerve.[55,58,59,62–64] Nerve conduction velocity and electromyography testing define the site and extent of injury.[56] MRI may be useful if a space-occupying mass or other anatomic variation within the anterior or lateral compartment of the leg is suspected to interrupt peroneal nerve conduction.[55]

Compression neuropathy of the posterior tibial nerve or its branches often mimics symptoms similar to CECS more than other compression neuropathies previously mentioned. Tarsal tunnel syndrome was first described in 2 separate investigations by Keck[65] and Lam[66] in 1962. Patients present with complaints of paresthesias, dysesthesias, or cramping along the plantar and less commonly the medial aspect of the foot. Symptoms increase with activity and remain for as little as 10 minutes or up to several hours. Patients may also complain of symptoms at night, a feature uncharacteristic of CECS.[67,68]

Clinical examination of tarsal tunnel syndrome frequently displays sensory and/or motor disturbances in the foot. An early sign of sensory loss is decreased 2-point discrimination on the medial and plantar aspects of the foot.[69,70] Over time, decreased perception of light touch and difficulties distinguishing sharp from dull in the plantar aspect of the foot are seen. Hypertrophy of the abductor hallucis may represent a site of nerve compression.[71] Patients with CECS will commonly present with symptoms localized to the abductor hallucis, simulating symptoms consistent with porta pedis or tarsal tunnel entrapment.

Several studies are used to determine the extent of nerve compression across the tarsal tunnel and calcaneal tunnels. Electrodiagnostic studies assess for neuropathic changes across the tarsal tunnel and porta pedis with a reported accuracy of 90%.[72] Although there are a number of different studies, the most sensitive are

1. Conduction velocities of the sensory nerves[72]
2. Motor evoked potentials to the abductor hallucis and abductor digiti minimi[73]
3. Electromyography of the abductor hallucis and abductor digiti minimi[74]

Use of all available tests is recommended. MRI assesses spatial relationships between anatomic components of the tarsal tunnel, as well as rules out the presence of space-occupying lesions.[75]

A review of the differential diagnosis for plantar foot pain would not be complete without mention of plantar fasciitis and heel pain syndrome.

Both are activity related; as intensity and duration increase, so will the symptoms. Patients with CECS frequently cannot continue their activity, but must stop for symptoms to resolve. Patients with heel pain syndrome or plantar fascitis are limited by their discomfort, but their pain does not commonly prevent them from continuing. Chronic heel pain and plantar fascitis respond consistently to conservative measures in up to 95% of cases.[76,77] Conservative management consists of casting,[78] night splints,[79] steroid injections,[80] rigid orthoses,[81] flexible orthoses,[82] nonsteroidal anti-inflammatory drugs,[83] stretching,[84] and the like. In contrast, CECS is not managed effectively with conservative measures alone.

DIAGNOSTIC TESTING PROCEDURES

Before proceeding with Intracompartmental Pressure Testing (ICPT), it is necessary to rule out vascular inflow conditions, which can create a similar clinical presentation.

Evaluating vascular supply is an integral part of the workup for CECS of the leg or foot. A Doppler examination can be performed before and after exercise to check for arterial inflow abnormalities. The patient also can be asked to plantarflex the foot while a Doppler is applied to the posterior tibial artery. A reduction or absence of flow during this maneuver may be a sign of popliteal artery entrapment syndrome. Alterations in Doppler flow during knee flexion may be a sign of popliteal adventitial cystic disease (Ishikawa maneuver).[49] An arterial segmental Doppler or arterial duplex Doppler can expose the location and extent of disease. The arterial segmental Doppler is performed at rest and after exercise that re-creates the patient's symptoms. Ideally, exercise should be continued until the patient experiences a maximal degree of symptoms or is forced to stop due to pain. The pre- and post-exercise ankle-brachial index should be nearly identical, with no reduction in pressure after exercise. A decrease in ankle-brachial index greater than 0.2 immediately after exercise is indicative of arterial inflow abnormality.[85] Pressures should return to baseline within 2 minutes. A return to baseline requiring 2 to 6 minutes may represent single-segment disease, and more than 6 minutes may indicate a multisegment inflow problem.[86] Arterial duplex Doppler provides an assessment of the internal quality and diameter of the vessel as well as flow velocity and degree of turbulent flow.[85] This is helpful in checking for arterial entrapment syndromes of the femoral and popliteal arteries. In cases in which flow abnormalities are demonstrated, an arteriogram would be the next step and a referral to a vascular surgeon may be needed.

Intracompartmental Pressure Testing

ICPT testing can be done statically, at rest or dynamically, during exercise, and after exercise. There are 2 systems that have been available for performing static intracompartmental testing. Both systems provide measurements in "mm Hg," are self-contained, and fairly easy to use. The 2 systems are (1) the Stryker IC System (Stryker Surgical, Kalamazoo, MI), and (2) the ACE IC system (ACE Medical Company, Los Angeles, CA). The Stryker IC System is no longer supported by the manufacturer, but new and used units may still be available for purchase online, along with sterile accessory kits.

It is paramount to follow a strict protocol if accurate measurements of the compartments of the foot are to be obtained. The patient should not perform any exercise on the day of testing. The patient is placed supine with a soft roll under both Achilles tendons. The elevation should not allow the calves to touch the table. The foot is allowed to passively relax into plantarflexion. The patient remains supine for 10 minutes to allow blood pressure stabilization. Two circles are drawn overlying the appropriate sites for measuring intracompartmental pressure. One site is used for obtaining the resting pressure. The second site is used to obtain the post-exercise pressure. A small volume of local anesthetic is infiltrated into the subcutaneous tissues superficial to the deep fascia to lessen the pain on catheter insertion. The device is calibrated according to the manufacturer's recommendations and the resting pressure is obtained. If multiple compartments are to be tested, resting pressures for each compartment are obtained, while the patient is at rest, before performing any exercise. The patient then performs an activity that will reproduce their symptoms until they can no longer continue. The patient quickly returns to their original position and undergoes post-exercise ICPT. Measurements are taken immediately on insertion of the catheter and every minute thereafter until 5 minutes have elapsed. In some cases, post-exercise pressures are taken every minute for 8 minutes to determine if they can return to their resting pressure. If another compartment of the foot needs to be tested, the patient performs the aggravating activity again until symptoms force the patient to stop and the procedure is repeated.

Catheter Insertion Sites for Intracompartmental Pressure Testing of the Foot

ICPT is primarily performed on the medial compartment, as it is most commonly involved in CECS of the foot. Nevertheless, it is helpful to have knowledge on where it is safe to test not only the medial, but also the superficial central, intermediate central/calcaneal, and lateral compartments. Reach and colleagues[87] used MRI to define the compartments of the foot as well as optimal needle placement and depth of insertion for ICPT. The medial compartment is tested from the medial side of the foot overlying the abductor hallucis at a point 60 mm directly inferior to the prominent point of the medial malleolus (**Figs. 1** and **2**). The needle is advanced laterally across the medial compartment to a depth of approximately 11 mm. The needle can then be advanced an additional 14 mm (total depth 25 mm) to enter the intermediate central compartment (calcaneal compartment - quadratus plantae). The insertion site for the lateral compartment can be found by locating the prominent aspect of the lateral malleolus and drawing a diagonal line toward the fifth metatarsal head and then going a distance of approximately 109 mm (in a proximal direction), in-line with the fifth ray. The needle is advanced approximately 11 mm to enter the lateral compartment (**Fig. 3**). In patients with a shorter foot, mark the proximal aspect of the styloid process of the fifth metatarsal, and the center of the fifth metatarsal head. The point of entrance into the lateral compartment is at the midpoint between the proximal and distal extent

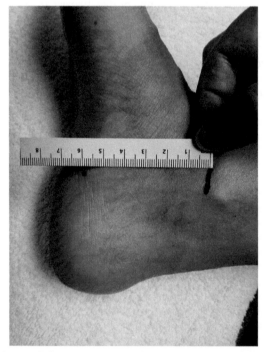

Fig. 1. ICPT for the medial compartment. The insertion point for testing the medial compartment is found by locating the most caudal point of the medial malleolus and measuring 50 to 60 mm directly inferior to a point overlying the abductor hallucis muscle.

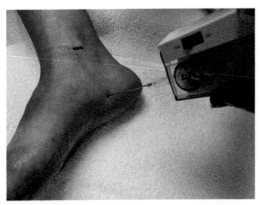

Fig. 2. ICPT for the medial compartment. The needle is then advanced to a depth of approximately 11 mm. To measure the intermediate central compartment (calcaneal compartment – quadratus plantae); continue to advance the needle to a depth of approximately 25 mm.

of the fifth metatarsal (**Figs. 4** and **5**). The needle is advanced approximately 11 mm to enter the lateral compartment. The superficial central compartment (flexor digitorum brevis) is measured from the plantar aspect of the foot. Locate the midpoint of the posterior aspect of the heel. Measure anteriorly 115 mm, staying central on the plantar foot. On reaching a point 115 mm from the start point, advance the needle approximately 11 mm to enter the superficial plantar compartment (**Figs. 6** and **7**).[87]

Criteria for Chronic Exertional Compartment Syndrome of the Foot

Normal resting compartment pressures should be less than 10 mm Hg.[88–91] Dayton and colleagues[88] measured resting pressures in the central fascial compartment of the foot in 25 healthy volunteers with a mean age of 42.2 years (range 15–72 years). Measurements were taken with an arterial line monitor and the Stryker Intracompartmental Pressure Device. The mean compartmental pressure value for the central fascial compartment was 4.69 ± 2.62 mm Hg. A resting pressure greater than 15 mm Hg is

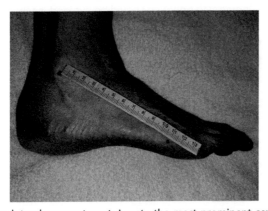

Fig. 3. ICPT for the lateral compartment. Locate the most prominent aspect of the lateral malleolus and draw a diagonal line toward the fifth metatarsal head and going a distance (in a proximal direction) of approximately 109 mm, in-line with the fifth ray, is the insertion point for testing the lateral compartment.

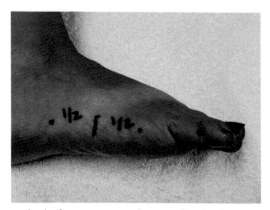

Fig. 4. Alternative method of measurement for ICPT for the lateral compartment. In patients with a shorter foot, mark the proximal aspect of the styloid process of the fifth metatarsal, and the center of the fifth metatarsal head. The point of entrance into the lateral compartment is at the midpoint between the proximal and distal extent of the fifth metatarsal.

suggestive (but not definitive) of CECS. A 1-minute post-exercise intracompartmental pressure reading greater than 30 mm Hg is highly suggestive of CECS of the foot.[92] A 5-minute post-exercise pressure reading greater than 20 mm Hg and/or a prolonged return to resting pressure between 8 and 15 minutes is also suggestive of CECS.[90,91,93]

TREATMENT
Conservative Care

Once a diagnosis of CECS of the foot has been made, treatment options can be entertained. Documentation in the world literature on conservative management for CECS of the foot is almost nonexistent. A fundamental option for conservative care is to limit the intensity and duration of offending activity or eliminate it altogether. If an individual wishes to continue activities that aggravate the condition, it is imperative to reduce external pressure. Shoegear should be in contact with the foot but not providing additional compression. Sockwear should not be constrictive. Compression garments should be avoided. Conforming orthotics should be avoided, as these devices provide

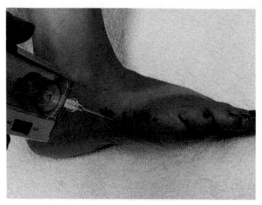

Fig. 5. Alternative method of measurement for ICPT for the lateral compartment. Insert the needle to a depth of approximately 11 mm.

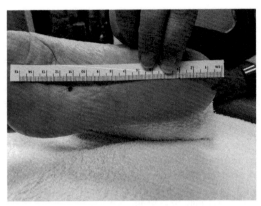

Fig. 6. ICPT for the superficial central compartment. Locate the midpoint of the posterior aspect of the heel and measure anteriorly approximately 115 mm, staying central on the plantar foot.

increased pressures to the plantar and plantarmedial aspects of the foot. Conservative management for CECS of the leg has Level IV evidence; some of these treatments may be helpful in CECS of the foot.

Blackman and colleagues[94] assessed the effects of a conservative treatment program in 7 patients with CECS of the anterior compartment. Participants received 6 treatments of massage to the anterior and posterior compartments of the leg by a

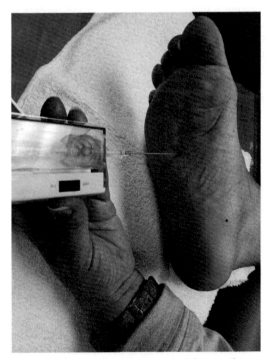

Fig. 7. ICPT for the superficial central compartment. Advance the needle to a depth of 11 mm.

physical therapist over 5 weeks. The participants were also instructed on how to stretch the anterior and posterior compartments of the leg twice a day. The investigators found no statistically significant difference in post-exercise anterior compartment pressures. There was a statistically significant reduction in pain after exercise following the treatment program. Furthermore, patients had a significantly greater amount of work output in dorsiflexion (tested isokinetically) following the massage and stretching intervention. The investigation used a limited number of patients, and patients received only 6 massage treatments over 5 weeks. A more common physical therapy program would involve 2 or 3 treatments per week for 4 to 6 weeks. It is conceivable that a greater number of treatments in conjunction with a home program (eg, foam rolling, aggressive soft tissue mobilization) could result in less pain and even greater work output. Altering loading patterns during walking and running has been used by several authors to reduce symptoms in the anterior compartment of the leg.[95–99] Many runners habitually heel strike, which places the knee in terminal extension and the ankle joint in excessive dorsiflexion at ground contact. This requires increased eccentric activity of the anterior compartment muscles to decelerate the foot to the ground. It is possible to train an individual to land foot flat at the time of initial contact. The process involves loading the foot under the center of mass and decreasing forward stride length by increasing cadence (180 steps/min). Pulling the foot off the ground with the hamstring muscles reduces push-off with the gastroc-soleus muscles. Altering walking or running patterns has not been proven to reduce muscle activity in the foot, thus lessening symptoms of CECS.

Conservative management of CECS of the foot is classically ineffective. Fascial decompression of the medial, central superficial, and lateral compartments is the most effective course of action. The approach to the medial and superficial central compartments is through a longitudinal curved incision centered over the abductor hallucis. The incision is deepened down to the superficial fascia of the abductor hallucis (**Figs. 8** and **9**). The superficial fascia will frequently be thinner overlying the muscle in the distal two-thirds and can be thicker in the proximal one-third of the incision. The superficial fascia is incised; if exceptionally thick, it can be partially excised. In some cases, the abductor hallucis is exceptionally hypertrophied or can have an accessory muscle belly.[100,101] The muscle can be debulked along its superficial aspect without compromising its functionality. The abductor hallucis is then elevated,

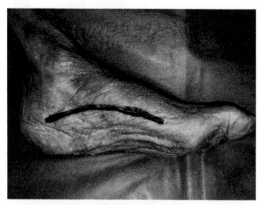

Fig. 8. A longitudinal curved incision is centered over the abductor hallucis muscle belly and deepened to the superficial fascia. The superficial fascia can be thicker proximally, but in most cases it is very thin overlying the abductor hallucis.

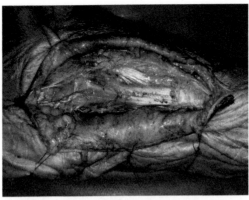

Fig. 9. The skin is tied back carefully, limiting tension on the margins of the incision. The superficial facia in this specimen is quite thin.

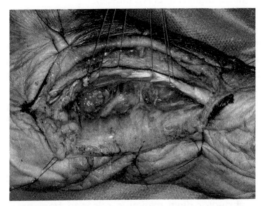

Fig. 10. The abductor hallucis muscle belly has been elevated allowing visualization of the medial intermuscular septum. In this specimen, the intermuscular septum is very thin and atrophic.

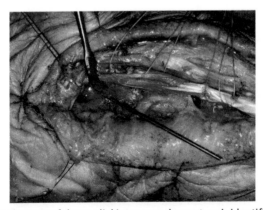

Fig. 11. The proximal aspect of the medial intermuscular septum is identified and a stab incision is made within the upper one-half, and opened from distal to proximal to enter the intermediate central compartment (calcaneal compartment – quadratus plantae). The probe is pointing at the distal portion of the quadratus plantae of the deep central compartment.

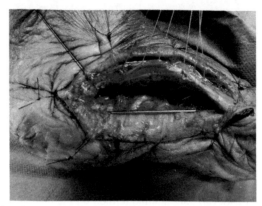

Fig. 12. A probe has been placed along the lower margin of the medial intermuscular septum. The septum is incised from proximal to distal to gain entrance into the superficial central compartment (flexor digitorum brevis muscle).

allowing visualization of the medial intermuscular septum (**Fig. 10**). The intermediate central compartment (quadratus plantae - calcaneal compartment) is entered by identifying the proximal aspect of the intermuscular septum deep to the abductor hallucis. A small incision is then made in the upper one-half of the septum with a surgical blade and the incision is extended with a Metzenbaum scissor from distal to proximal. It will be possible to identify the distal portion of the quadratus plantae[10] (**Fig. 11**). It should be noted that the lateral plantar nerve (and its branches), artery, and accompanying veins are in close proximity. To enter the superficial central compartment, the lower margin of the medial intermuscular septum is incised from proximal to distal, providing entrance into the flexor digitorum brevis (**Figs. 12** and **13**). In rare cases, a patient will present with CECS of the lateral compartment of the foot. The lateral compartment is addressed through a lateral linear incision overlying the abductor digiti minimi. The fascia overlying the abductor digiti minimi is released from proximal to distal. On completion of fascial decompression(s), subcutaneous tissues and skin are closed in a standard manner over a suction drain. The drain can be removed 48 to 72 hours after surgery. The patient is placed in a Jones compression dressing or bi-valved

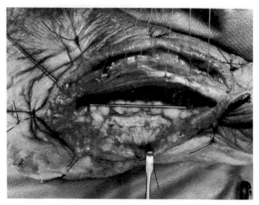

Fig. 13. The fascia overlying the superficial central compartment has been incised and reflected. The probe is lying on the reflected fascia. The flexor digitorum brevis and the underlying plantar fascia can be seen below the probe.

below-the-knee fiberglass cast for 2 weeks while non-weightbearing. The patient advances into a removable cast boot and partial weightbearing between weeks 2 and 4. Physical therapy can begin after week 2 and will involve soft tissue mobilization to the medial and plantar arches and leg, and open chain strengthening. Weightbearing as tolerated begins after week 4. Closed chain strengthening advances as tolerated. Return to sport varies, but usually does not begin until week 10 to 12.

SUMMARY

CECS of the foot is considered a rare cause of medial arch and heel pain. It may actually be more common, but is overlooked because of its unusual presentation and response to conservative care. Patients experience pain in the medial or proximal arch/heel aggravated by taping or orthotics, interventions classically effective for plantar fascial or arch-related conditions. Unlike patients with plantar fasciitis, posterior tibial tendon disorders, or other arch-related conditions, there is no tenderness over the plantar fascia, at the insertion of the posterior tibial tendon or along the tendon itself. Post-exercise examination reveals tenderness over the abductor hallucis and diffuse plantar central arch tenderness if the superficial central compartment is involved. Confirming a diagnosis of CECS is achieved with intracompartmental pressure testing, assuming there are no vascular inflow abnormalities. Conservative care is frequently ineffective, and open release of the involved compartments (primarily medial and superficial central) is often required.

CLINICS CARE POINTS

- Patients with CECS of the foot typically experience pain within the medial, plantar central, or plantar medial proximal arch with activity. Orthotics, arch taping, or compression garments will usually aggravate their symptoms.

- Abnormalities in arterial inflow can mimic symptoms consistent with CECS of the foot. It is helpful to perform either an arterial segmental Doppler examination, an arterial duplex scan, or an arteriogram to define the level and extent of arterial embarrassment in the limb.

- ICPT is critically important in establishing a diagnosis of CECS of the foot. Resting compartment pressures should be less than 10 mm Hg. A 1-minute post-exercise pressure greater than 30 mm Hg is diagnostic for CECS of the foot.

- The medial and superficial central compartments of the foot are most commonly involved in CECS of the foot. A surgical release of the abductor hallucis muscle through a curved longitudinal incision is generally curative.

ACKNOWLEDGMENTS

The author would like to thank Richard T. Bouché, DPM, and Chad L. Seidenstricker, DPM for their assistance with the manuscript.

DISCLOSURE

The author has nothing to disclose as it relates to this subject matter.

REFERENCES

1. Freedman BJ. Dr. Edward Wilson of the Antarctic; a biographical sketch, followed by an inquiry into the nature of his last illness. Proc R Soc Med 1953; 47:7.

2. Horn CE. Acute ischemia of the anterior tibial muscle and the long extensor muscles of the toes. J Bone Joint Surg 1945;27A:615–22.
3. Mavor GE. The anterior tibial syndrome. J Bone Joint Surg 1956;38A:513–7.
4. Bouche RT. Chronic compartment syndrome of the leg. J Am Podiatr Med Assoc 1990;80(12):633–48.
5. Lokiec F, Siev-Ner I, Pritsch M. Chronic compartment syndrome of both feet. J Bone Joint Surg Br 1991;73:178–9.
6. Seiler R, Guziec G. Chronic compartment syndrome of the foot - a case report. J Am Podiatr Med Assoc 1994;84:91–4.
7. Muller GP, Masquelet AC. Chronic compartment syndrome of the foot: a case report. Rev Chir Orthop Reparatrice Appar Mot 1995;81:549–52.
8. Mollica MB. Chronic exertional compartment syndrome of the foot: a case report. J Am Podiatr Med Assoc 1998;88:21–4.
9. Jowett A, Birks C, Blackney M. Chronic exertional compartment syndrome in the medial compartment of the foot. Foot Ankle Int 2008;29(8):838–41.
10. Izadi FE, Richie DH Jr. Exertional compartment syndrome of the medial foot compartment – diagnosis and treatment: a case report. J Am Podiatr Med Assoc 2014;104(4):417–21.
11. Sinikumpu JJ, Lepojärvi S, Serlo W, et al. Atraumatic compartment syndrome of the foot in a 15-year-old female. J Foot Ankle Surg 2013;52(1):72–5.
12. Park YH, Ahn JH, Choi GW, et al. Exertional medial compartment syndrome of the foot: referred pain and sequelae of delayed diagnosis – a case report. Clin J Sport Med 2019;29(6):e83–5.
13. Amendola A, Rorbeck CH, Vellett D, et al. The use of magnetic resonance imaging in exertional compartment syndromes. Am J Sports Med 1990;18(1):29–34.
14. Dahl M, Hansen P, Stal P, et al. Stiffness and thickness of fascia do not explain chronic exertional compartment syndrome. Clin Orthop Relat Res 2011;469:3495–500.
15. Eaton RG, Green WT. Epimysiotomy and fasciotomy in the treatment of Volkman's ischemic contracture. Orthop Clin North Am 1972;3:175–86.
16. Burton AC. On the physical equilibrium of small blood vessels. Am J Physiol 1951;164:319–29.
17. Ashton H. The effect of increased tissue pressure on blood flow. Clin Orthop Relat Res 1975;113:15–26.
18. Ashton H. Critical closing pressure in human peripheral vascular beds. Clin Sci 1962;22:79–87.
19. Hargens AR, Mubarak SJ, Akeson WH. Current concepts in the pathophysiology, evaluation and diagnosis of compartment syndrome. Hand Clin 1998;14:371–83.
20. Matsen FA III, Winquist RA, Krugmire RB Jr. Diagnosis and management of compartmental syndromes. J Bone Joint Surg Am 1980;62:286–91.
21. Draves DJ. Anatomy of the lower extremity. Baltimore (MD): Williams & Wilkins; 1986. p. 291–301.
22. Woodburne RT. Essentials of human anatomy. 6th edition. New York: Oxford University Press; 1978. p. 573–82.
23. Goss CM. Gray's anatomy. Philadelphia: Lea and Febiger; 1973. p. 355–9.
24. Grodinsky M. A study of the fascial spaces of the foot and their bearing on infections. Surg Gynecol Obstet 1929;49:737–51.
25. Feingold ML, Resnick D, Niwayama G, et al. The plantar compartments of the foot: a roentgen approach. I. Experimental observations. Invest Radiol 1977;12:281–8.

26. Myerson MS. Acute compartment syndromes of the foot. Bull Hosp Jt Dis Orthop Inst 1987;47:251–61.
27. Myerson MS. Experimental decompression of the fascial compartments of the foot - the basis for fasciotomy in acute compartment syndromes. Foot Ankle 1988;8:308–14.
28. Myerson M. Diagnosis and treatment of compartment syndrome of the foot. Orthopedics 1990;13:711–7.
29. Manoli A II, Weber TG. Fasciotomy of the foot - an anatomical study with special reference to release of the calcaneal compartment. Foot Ankle 1990;10:267–75.
30. Sarrafian SK. Anatomy of the foot and ankle. Philadelphia: J. B. Lippincott; 1993. p. 149–58.
31. Martin BF. Observations on the muscles and tendons of the medial aspect of the sole of the foot. J Anat 1964;98:437–53.
32. Goldman F. Deep space infections in the diabetic patient. J Am Podiatr Med Assoc 1987;8:431–43.
33. Kamel R, Sakla FB. Anatomical compartments of the sole of the human foot. Anat Rec 1961;140:57–60.
34. Goodwin DW, Salonen DC, Yu JS, et al. Plantar compartments of the foot: MR appearance in cadavers and diabetic patients. Radiology 1995;196:623–30.
35. Levin J, Zier BG, Grandinetti GM, et al. Peripheral vascular disease. In: Zier BG, editor. Essentials of internal medicine in clinical podiatry. Philadelphia: WB Saunders; 1990. p. 74–81.
36. Jones RO. Podiatric implications of popliteal artery entrapment syndrome. J Am Podiatr Med Assoc 1986;76:20–2.
37. McDonald PT, Easterbrook JA, Rich NM, et al. Popliteal artery entrapment. Am J Surg 1980;139:318–25.
38. Rich NM, Collins GJ, McDonald PT, et al. Popliteal vascular entrapment. Arch Surg 1979;114:1377–84.
39. Love JW, Whelan TJ. Popliteal artery entrapment syndrome. Am J Surg 1965; 109:620–4.
40. Insua JA, Young JR, Humphries AW. Popliteal artery entrapment syndrome. Arch Surg 1970;101:771–5.
41. Whelan TJ Jr. Popliteal artery entrapment. In: Haimoviei H, editor. Vascualr surgery. New York: McGraw-Hill; 1976. p. 493–504.
42. Ferrero R, Barile C, Buzzacchino A, et al. La sindrome da costrizione dell'arteria poplitea. Minerva Cardioangiol 1978;26:389–410.
43. Leu HJ, Odermatt B. Pathogenesis of the so-called cystic adventitial degeneration of peripheral blood vessels. Virchows Arch 1984;404:289–300.
44. Ejurp B, Hierton T. Intermittent claudication: three cases treated by a free vein graft. Acta Chir Scand 1954;108:217–30.
45. Ruppell V, Sperling M, Schott KE. Pathologisch-anatomische boebachtungen bie zystischer adventitiadegeneration der blutgefaBe. Beitr Pathol 1971;144: 101–12.
46. Sys J, Michielsen J, Bleyn J, et al. Adventitial cystic disease of the popliteal artery in a triathlete. Am J Sports Med 1997;25:854–7.
47. Donayre CE. Adventitial cystic disease. In: White RA, Hollier LH, editors. Vascular surgery: basic science and clinical correlations. Philadelphia: JB Lippincott; 1994. p. 199–205.
48. Ward AS, Reidy JF. Case report: adventitial cystic disease of the popliteal artery. Clin Radiol 1987;38:649–51.

49. Ishikawa K, Mishima Y, Kobayashi S. Cystic adventitial disease of the popliteal artery: report of a case. Angiology 1961;12:357–66.

50. Lee BY, LaPointe DG, Madden JL. The adductor canal syndrome. Am J Surg 1972;123:617–20.

51. Balaji MR, DeWeese JA. Adductor canal outlet syndrome. JAMA 1981;245:167–70.

52. Gray H. The arteries of the lower limb. In: Goss CM, editor. Gray's anatomy. 29th edition. Philadelphia: Lea & Febiger; 1973. p. 656–7.

53. Henry AK. Extensile exposure. Edinburgh (London): E & S Livingstone; 1945. p. 163.

54. Adkison DP, Bosse MJ, Gaccione DR, et al. Anatomical variations in the course of the superficial peroneal nerve. J Bone Joint Surg 1991;73:112–4.

55. Daghino W, Pasquali M, Faletti C. Superficial peroneal nerve entrapment in a young athlete: the diagnostic contribution of magnetic resonance imaging. J Foot Ankle Surg 1997;36:170–2.

56. Styf J. Entrapment of the superficial peroneal nerve. J Bone Joint Surg 1989;71:131–5.

57. Garfin S, Mubarak SJ, Owen CA. Exertional anterolateral- compartment syndrome. J Bone Joint Surg 1977;59:404–5.

58. Leach RE, Purnell MB, Saito A. Peroneal nerve entrapment in runners. Am J Sports Med 1989;17:287–91.

59. Lowdon IMR. Superficial peroneal nerve entrapment. J Bone Joint Surg Br 1985;67:58–9.

60. McAuliffe TB, Fiddian NJ, Browett JP. Entrapment neuropathy of the superficial peroneal nerve. J Bone Joint Surg 1985;67:62–3.

61. Kopell HP, Thompson WAL. Peripheral entrapment neuropathies. Baltimore (MD): Williams and Wilkins; 1963.

62. Banerjee T, Koons DD. Superficial peroneal nerve entrapment: report of two cases. J Neurosurg 1981;55:991–2.

63. Kernohan J, Levack B, Wilson JN. Entrapment of the superficial peroneal nerve. J Bone Joint Surg 1985;67:60–1.

64. Styf J, Morberg P. The superficial peroneal tunnel syndrome. J Bone Joint Surg 1997;79:801–3.

65. Keck C. The tarsal-tunnel syndrome. J Bone Joint Surg 1962;44:180–2.

66. Lam SJS. A tarsal tunnel syndrome. Lancet 1962;2:1354–5.

67. Pfeiffer WH, Cracchiolo A. Clinical results after tarsal tunnel decompression. J Bone Joint Surg 1994;76:1222–30.

68. Turan I, Rivero-Melian C, Gunter P, et al. Tarsal tunnel syndrome. Clin Orthop Relat Res 1997;343:152–6.

69. Tassler PA, Dellon AL. Correlation of measurements of pressure perception using the pressure-specified sensory device with electrodiagnostic testing. J Occup Med 1995;37:862–6.

70. Tassleer PL, Dellon AL. Pressure perception in the normal lower extremity and in the tarsal tunnel syndrome. Muscle Nerve 1996;19:285–9.

71. Pace N, Serafini P, Iacono EL, et al. The tarsal and calcaneal tunnel syndromes. J Orthop Traumatol 1991;17:247–52.

72. Galardi G, Amadio S, Maderna L, et al. Electrophysiologic studies in tarsal tunnel syndrome: diagnostic reliability of motor distal latency, mixed nerve and sensory nerve conduction velocities. Am J Phys Med Rehabil 1994;73:193–8.

73. Kaplan PE, Kernahan WT. Tarsal tunnel syndrome: an electrodiagnostic and surgical correlation. J Bone Joint Surg 1981;63:96–9.

74. Fu R, Delisa JA, Kraft GH. Motor nerve latencies through the tarsal tunnel in normal adult subjects: standard determinations corrected for temperature and distance. Arch Phys Med Rehabil 1994;73:193–8.

75. Frey C, Kerr R. Magnetic resonance imaging and the evaluation of tarsal tunnel syndrome. Foot Ankle 1993;14:159–64.

76. Bordelon RL. Heel pain. In: Mann RA, editor. Surgery of the foot and ankle, ed. 6. St Louis (MO): CV Mosby; 1993. p. 837–47.

77. Davis PF, Severud E, Baxter DE. Painful heel syndrome: results of nonoperative treatment. Foot Ankle Int 1994;15:531–5.

78. Tisdel CL, Harper M. Chronic plantar heel pain: treatment with a short leg walking cast. Foot Ankle Int 1996;17:41–2.

79. Wapner K, Sharkey PF. The use of night splints for treatment of recalcitrant plantar fasciitis. Foot Ankle 1991;12:135–7.

80. Lutter LD. Surgical decisions in athletes' subcalcaneal pain. Am J Sports Med 1986;14:481–5.

81. O'Brien D, Martin WJ. A retrospective analysis of heel pain. J Am Podiatr Med Assoc 1985;75:416–8.

82. Snider MP, Clancy WG, McBeath AA. Plantar fascia release for chronic plantar fasciitis in runners. Am J Sports Med 1983;11:215–9.

83. Snook GA, Chrisman OD. The management of subcalcaneal pain. Clin Orthop 1972;28:163–8.

84. Schepsis AA, Leach RE, Gorzyca J. Plantar fasciitis etiology, treatment, surgical and review of the literature. Clin Orthop 1991;266:185–96.

85. Sibley RC, Reis SP, MacFarlane JJ, et al. Non-invasive vascular studies: a guide to diagnosing peripheral arterial disease. Radiographics 2017;37(1):346–57.

86. Mohler ER 3rd. Peripheral arterial disease: identification and implications. Arch Intern Med 2003;163(19):2306–14.

87. Reach JS Jr, Amrami KK, Felmlee JP, et al. The compartments of the foot: a 3-Tesla magnetic resonance imaging study with clinical correlates for needle pressure testing. Foot Ankle Int 2007;28(5):584–94.

88. Dayton P, Goldman FD, Barton E. Compartment pressure in the foot: analysis of normal values and measurement technique. J Am Podiatr Med Assoc 1990; 80(10):521–5.

89. Murbarak SJ, Hargens AR, Owen CA, et al. The wick catheter technique for measurement of intramuscular pressure. J Bone Joint Surg 1976;58A:1016–20.

90. Mollica MB, Duyshart SC. Analysis of pre- and postexercise compartment pressures in the medial compartment of the foot. Am J Sports Med 2002;30(2): 268–71.

91. Pedowitz RA, Hargens AR, Mubarek SJ, et al. Modified criteria for the objective diagnosis of chronic compartment syndrome of the leg. Am J Sports Med 1990; 18(1):35–40.

92. Aweid O, Del Buono A, Malliaras P, et al. Systematic review and recommendations for intracompartment pressure monitoring in diagnosing chronic exertional compartment syndrome. Clin J Sport Med 2012;22(4):356–70.

93. Rorabeck CH, Bourne RB, Fowler PJ, et al. The role of tissue pressure measurements in diagnosing chronic anterior compartment syndrome. Am J Sports Med 1988;16(2):143–6.

94. Blackman PG, Simmons L,R, Crossley KM. Treatment of chronic exertional anterior compartment syndrome with massage: a pilot study. Clin J Sport Med 1998; 8(1):14–7.

95. Zimmermann WO, Bakker EWP. Reducing vertical ground reaction forces: the relative importance of three gait retraining cues. Clin Biomech (Bristol, Avon) 2019;69:16–20.

96. Zimmermann WO, Hutchinson M,R, Van den Berg R, et al. Conservative treatment of anterior chronic exertional compartment syndrome in the military, with a mid-term follow-up. BMJ Open Sport Exerc Med 2019;5(1):e000532.

97. Helmhout P,H, Diebal A,R, van der Kaaden L, et al. The effectiveness of a 6-week intervention program aimed at modifying running style in patients with chronic exertional compartment syndrome: results from a series of case studies. Orthop J Sports Med 2015;3(3). 2325967115575691.

98. Diebal AR, Gregory R, Alitz C, et al. Forefoot running improves pain and disability associated with chronic exertional compartment syndrome. Am J Sports Med 2012;40(5):1060–7.

99. Diebal AR, Gregory R, Alitz C, et al. Effects of forefoot running on chronic exertional compartment syndrome: a case series. Int J Sports Phys Ther 2011;6(4): 312–21.

100. Bhansali R,M, Bhansali R,R. Accessory abductor hallucis causing entrapment of the posterior tibial nerve. J Bone Joint Surg Br 1987;69(3):479–80.

101. Haber J,A, Sollitto R,J. Accessory abductor hallucis: a case report. J Foot Surg 1979;18(2):74–6.

Differentiating Achilles Insertional Calcific Tendinosis and Haglund's Deformity

Sean T. Grambart, DPM[a,b,]*, Jay Lechner, BS[a], Jennifer Wentz, BS[a]

KEYWORDS

- Haglund's • Achilles insertional calcific tendinosis • Achilles calcification
- Achilles calcific tendinitis • Pump bump

KEY POINTS

- There is a differentiation between Haglund's deformity and Achilles insertional calcific tendinosis.
- Surgical management of Achilles insertional calcific tendinosis involves detachment and reattachment of the Achilles tendon, whereas the majority of the Achilles tendon does not need detachment in a Haglund's.
- Postoperative recovery varies between Achilles insertional calcific tendinosis and Haglund's deformity.

INTRODUCTION

Calcaneodynia (heel pain) is an extremely common cause of foot pain. Approximately 15% of patients will experience some sort of heel pain.[1–5] The differential diagnoses for heel pain are extensive and can be broken down into the broad categories of soft tissue, osseous, infectious, and systemic pathologies. Soft tissue pathologies include ligament and tendon pathology, bursitis, plantar fasciitis, plantar fasciosis, plantar fascia tears, tarsal tunnel syndrome, neuroma, fat pad atrophy, plantar fibromatosis, and plantar fascia xanthoma. Osseous pathology includes calcaneal fracture, os trigonum syndrome, myositis or tendinitis, ossificans traumatic, osteoma, osteoarthritis, osteomyelitis, bone cyst, bone tumors, periostitis, bone bruise, osteochondral defect, Sever's disease, and Haglund's pathology. Some pathology, like Achilles insertional calcific tendinosis (AICT), involves both the soft tissue and osseous categories. Infectious sources include *Mycobacterium tuberculosis*, gonorrhea, syphilis, and bacterial infection.

[a] Des Moines University, College of Podiatric Medicine and Surgery, 3200 Grand Avenue, Des Moines, IA 50312, USA; [b] Unitypoint Health – Iowa Methodist Medical Center, Des Moines, IA, USA
* Corresponding author. 3200 Grand Avenue, Des Moines, IA 50312.
E-mail address: Sean.Grambart@dmu.edu

Clin Podiatr Med Surg 38 (2021) 165–181
https://doi.org/10.1016/j.cpm.2020.12.003
0891-8422/21/© 2020 Elsevier Inc. All rights reserved.

podiatric.theclinics.com

Systemic causes include Reiter's syndrome, rheumatoid arthritis, ankylosing spondylitis, psoriatic arthritis, reactive arthritis, gout, calcium pyrophosphate dihydrate deposition, fibromyalgia, steroid use, and oral fluoroquinolone.[1,3,5–19]

The large number of possible pathologies inherently leads to a large number of differential diagnosis and some confusion on terminology. Accurate diagnosis can be made from a thorough history and physical examination and imaging including use of radiographs, MRI, computed tomography scans, high-frequency ultrasound, and laboratory tests.[1,3–6,19–21] The purpose of this article is to discuss 2 very common causes of posterior and lateral heel pain: AICT and Haglund's deformity.

PERTINENT ANATOMY

The calcaneus is the largest and strongest tarsal bone in the foot with an average anterior to posterior length of 75 to 89 mm.[1,22] The posterior dorsal third of the calcaneus has the posterior facet that the talus articulates with and forms 1 of 3 articular surfaces for the subtalar joint. The lateral surface of the calcaneus can have 3 distinct prominences: retrotrochlear eminence, peroneal trochlea, and the third tubercle. The most distinguishing feature on the medial surface is the sustentaculum tali. The plantar surface of the calcaneus has 2 distinct landmarks, namely, the anterior tubercle and the calcaneal tuberosity, which is composed of a medial and lateral processes with an intermediate depression.[15] The posterior surface can be separated into 2 main parts. The superior aspect is a smooth, triangular-shaped surface for the bursa and its respective oval facet.[1,23] The middle aspect is a rough quadrilateral surface for the attachment of the Achilles tendon.[9]

The gastrocnemius muscle has 2 muscle bellies that originate from both the medial and lateral femoral condyles posteriorly and the medial adductor tubercle.[24] The soleus lies anterior to the gastrocnemius and originates from the soleal line on the posterior tibia, fibula, and interosseous membrane.[1,24] Together, these 2 muscles unite distally to form the Achilles tendon, which can also be referred to as the triceps surae.[25] The Achilles tendon is approximately 15 cm long and is composed of type 1 collagen, elastin, and proteoglycan.[26,27] The fibers of the Achilles tendon spiral counterclockwise approximately 90° with a range of 30° to 150° as the tendon moves from proximal to distal.[24,28–30] The tendon inserts obliquely to the calcaneus and forms an acute angle that fits it in tight proximity in a concave fashion along the calcaneus.[1,23] A normal Achilles tendon should be less than 10 mm thick in the anterior to posterior direction.[13] The Achilles tendon lacks a tendon sheath in the traditional sense and instead has a paratenon that surrounds the tendon.[1] The 2 layers of the paratenon consist of a visceral layer and a parietal layer. Aside from the gliding of the tendon in the paratenon, the paratenon plays another significant role. The tendon receives some vascular input from the anterior Kager's triangle, the myotenindous junction, and the attachment into the calcaneus, but the paratenon is its main vascular supply.[4,24,31,32] Although this layer supplies the tendon with the majority of its blood supply, the vascularity will decrease with age and lead to a critical zone of hypovascularity 2 to 6 cm above its insertion at the calcaneus.[1,26,33]

Patrik Haglund noticed 2 bursae in the posterior heel, which he named bursa achillea inferior–posterior and bursa achillea superior–anterior.[14] The bursas are lined with synovial fluid and exist to decrease mechanical friction.[15,16] Today, the bursas have different names. Between the posterior superior portion of the calcaneus and the Achilles tendon lies a disk, saddle-shaped, or horseshoe-shaped bursa named the retrocalcaneal bursa or the pre-Achilles bursa.[17,34] This bursa has fibrocartilage anteriorly; the posterior bursa blends with the paratenon.[23,24,35] The second bursa lies between the midline or slightly lateral to the Achilles tendon and the posterior subcutaneous tissue named the retro-Achilles bursa or superficial tendo Achilles bursa.[15,17,36,37] This bursa is present more during pathologic times, leading to inflammation of the bursa.[1] Usually, deep bursas such as the retrocalcaneal bursa are present at birth, whereas the superficial bursas like the retro-Achilles bursa is not always present at birth and develops owing to friction.[38,39] Typically, a nonpathologic bursa in the posterior heel measures 1 mm anterior to posterior, less than 7 mm proximal to distal, and less than 11 mm from medial to lateral. If the bursa measures larger than these given values, the bursa is usually pathologic.[34,35]

HAGLUND'S DEFORMITY

Patrik Haglund contributed greatly to the advancement of medicine throughout his career. He was born in 1870 in Norrköping, Sweden. Haglund studied under an orthopedic surgeon who had a special interest in extremity medicine, which led him into orthopedic medicine. In 1903, he completed his doctoral thesis looking at cancellous bone in the calcaneus and its functional structure through radiographs. One of his monumental works from 1927 is attributed to be the first clinical case in a 20-year-old woman with what would eventually be called Haglund's syndrome.[14,17] In this original article, the radiographs did not indicate any calcification across the posterior insertion. The term Haglund's prominence and deformity was not coined until 1982 by Pavlov and 1984 by Vega when they gave credit to Haglund, respectively.[15,30,39,40]

Starting in the 1990s, many analogies were then used to describe Haglund's pathology: pump bump, winter heel, retrocalcaneal exostosis, Mulholland's deformity, knobby heels, calcaneal altus, highbown heel, Albert's disease, policeman's heel, Achilles bursitis, retrocalcaneal bursitis, and prow beak, and in the Caribbean they use the term cucumber heel.[3,16,39,41] Within the Haglund definitions, the literature has used Haglund's disease, deformity, exostosis, syndrome, and triad. Owing to all of the variability and confusing nature of these terms, some authors have proposed to stop using all the analogies altogether (van Dijk and colleagues[39]). We believe that it is of the utmost importance to clarify the common analogies.

The term pump bump was initially introduced by Dickinson and Woodward in 1954.[42] This entity is the palpable soft tissue swelling seen with an inflamed bursa. The soft tissue is usually enlarged on the posterior superior-lateral aspect proximal to the Achilles insertion. Pump bump has been more associated with a systemic inflammatory disease.[4,15,39,40,43] Winter heel was coined by Nisbet in 1954 owing to the observation that the condition reoccurs during the winter season.[23,25] Haglund's deformity or exostosis is the prominent hypertrophic ovoid-, boat-, or tear-shaped bursal bony projections on the posterior superior-lateral calcaneus.[1,16,21,39,44]

Clinical Presentation

The most common patient population affected are women between the ages of 20 and 30 years.[3,10,15,19,23,40,45,46] Haglund's pathology can present unilaterally or bilaterally. Athletes such as runners are significantly affected owing to uphill training requiring maximum dorsiflexion.[1,12,23,25]

There are many theories regarding the cause of Haglund's deformity. Haglund postulated that the cultured man was more prone to developing Haglund's deformity and syndrome owing to wearing shoes.[14] Ill-fitting posterior shoe counters causes a higher mechanical pressure on the Achilles tendon and bursa from impingement of the soft tissue on the bursal projection.[1,15,16,40,45] Biomechanical theories discuss forces that lead to an increase in the calcaneal inclination angle by placing the calcaneus and bursal projection more vertical and, therefore, placing greater mechanical stress on the posterior lateral calcaneus and the soft tissue bursas. Many causes have been hypothesized, such as compensated rearfoot varus, compensated forefoot valgus, plantarflexed first ray, cavus foot, tibial varum, limited motion and more oblique subtalar joint axis, excessive frontal plane motion, excessive protonation, limb length discrepancy, vascular compromise, various shapes of the calcaneus, apophysitis during childhood, and trauma.[3,5,15,17,23,25,29,30,36,43–47]

Most patients with symptomatic Haglund's syndrome complain of acute or chronic posterior-lateral heel dull or achy pain, erythema, and possible edema that is worse while wearing shoes and with activity. Most pain occurs during heel strike and maximum dorsiflexion, which explains the increasing pain with sport.[5,16,35] This area may have a visual prominence, which is the spot that is tender to palpation[22] (**Fig. 1**). Discoloration and callusing of the skin can be present from shoe friction. One of the key factors with Haglund's deformity is that the Achilles tendon usually does not show any pathology and is asymptomatic when specifically palpating the tendon.

ACHILLES INSERTIONAL CALCIFIC TENDINOSIS

AICT is an Achilles pathology arising at the insertion of the tendon at the middle aspect of the posterior calcaneus. As the name indicates, this process also involves varying levels of mucoid degeneration of the tendon at or just proximal to the insertion site. Pain is a gradual onset that is usually seen middle age and typically present with midline tenderness to palpation of the tendon's complete insertion with a palpable calcification at the insertion (**Fig. 2**). In patients who are symptomatic with this condition, calcification of the distal tendon has been found to be more common.[44] Pain is

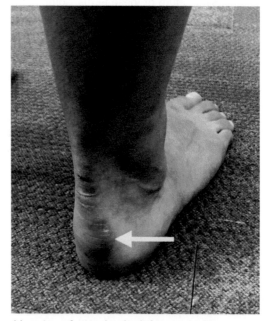

Fig. 1. Posterolateral location of a Haglund's deformity (*yellow arrow*).

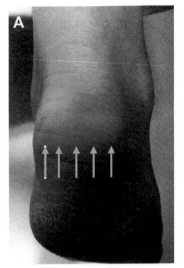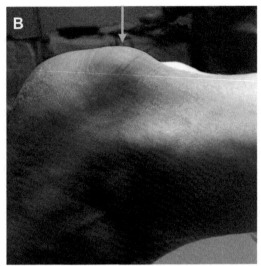

Fig. 2. (*A*) AICT expanding across the entire posterior aspect of the calcaneus (*green arrows*). (*B*) Posterior location of the AICT at the attachment site of the Achilles tendon (*green arrow*).

aggravated with activity and with shoes that have a heel counter. Further clinical findings include pain and swelling of the Achilles tendon just proximal to the insertion. Whereas in Haglund's deformity patients are young and active, patients with AICT have a tendency to be older and have a higher body mass index.

Several factors have been associated with the development of AICT. Equinus is common in these patients and one thought is the pull of the Achilles tendon at the insertion site from the equinus will form the calcification owing to Wolfe's law. In addition, various arthropathies have been associated with an increased incidence of calcification at the Achilles tendon insertion. Resnick and colleagues[48] retrospectively compared the heel radiographs of 100 patients with rheumatoid and variant arthropathies and compared them to a cohort of 75 patients without the arthropathies. Upon evaluation, they found that the incidence of posterior calcaneal spurring to be 11% in the control group and up to 56% in patients with underlying rheumatologic disorders.[48]

Histologic evaluation of the pathologic tendon reveals several morphologic changes. Ossification of the entheseal fibrocartilage, mucoid degeneration, necrosis, and hemorrhage are common findings.[49] In a study evaluating histologic specimens from 36 operations, Johansson and colleagues[20] found that the calcifications all had trabecular bone and medullary cavities resembling fetal mesenchymal tissue. It has also been found that the samples contained a large amount of fibrocartilage and diffusely organized chondrocytes within a collagen-rich medium. In a addition, within the histologic findings there is often an absence of inflammatory cells, leading to the proposal that AICT be referred to as a tendinosis rather than a tendinitis.[39]

IMAGING

Radiographic evaluation is a common step in the workup of the patient presenting with posterior heel pain. Several different angles and markings on a lateral radiograph have been used for the evaluation of Haglund's deformity. The Fowler–Phillip angle was first identified in 1945 and is formed from a line tangential to the posterosuperior surface of the bursal projection and greater tuberosity and a line tangential to the plantar calcaneal border[50] (**Fig. 3**). A normal value for the Fowler–Phillip angle is between 44° and 69°. This angle has been found to not be very useful as a prognostic measure by several authors, with a false-negative rate ranging from 86% to 100%.[15,29,46,51] Building on this angle, the total angle of Ruch includes the calcaneal inclination with the Fowler–Phillip angle. The total angle has been found to be marginally better than the Fowler–Phillip, with a sensitivity of 7.04% and false negative rate of 98.6%.[51] Parallel pitch lines are a measurement with a lower line formed from the calcaneal pitch and an upper line parallel from the posterior lip of the talar articular surface.[15] With the parallel pitch lines, a bursal or posterosuperior crest projection above the superior line is considered pathologic. The usefulness of this measure is mixed, with several authors finding an accuracy between 63.3% and 70.0% with false-negative rates between 30.0% to 36.7%, whereas others have found no significant difference between patients experiencing symptoms and those who are asymptomatic.[15,44,51,52]

Despite these angles not bearing strong diagnostic use, there are radiographic signs that may be more useful. The Chauvex–Liet angle, on a lateral view, is formed from the difference between the calcaneal pitch and an angle formed from the vertical of the most superior point of the great tuberosity of the calcaneus and a straight line from this point to the apex of the posterosuperior crest and is considered abnormal if the value is greater than between 10° and 12°.[53] This measurement has been identified by the original authors of having a sensitivity of 85% and by Singh and colleagues[51] at 73% for Haglund's deformity.[53]

The AICT will show a calcification, producing a step in the middle of the posterior surface of the calcaneus, and has been found to be significantly associated with symptomatic patients.[29,44,51] Research has also shown that more than 70% of patients with insertional tendinitis symptoms have calcifications of the tendon visible

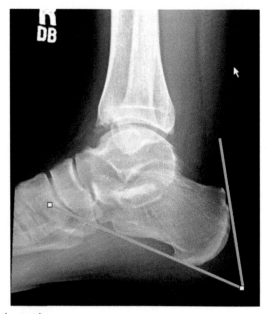

Fig. 3. Phillip–Fowler angle.

on radiographs.[44,52] Calcifications within the tendon itself are also a common finding in patients suffering from insertional tendonitis and posterior heel pain, being identified in 73% of patients by Kang and colleagues[52] and 78.4% of patients by Lu and colleagues.[44] This calcification can easily be seen on the lateral view (**Fig. 4**), but the oblique view can be used to evaluate the extent of the calcification from medial to lateral, which is important in differentiating Haglund's deformity as well as for preoperative planning (**Fig. 5**).

Although the clinical symptoms and plain radiograph findings can lead to the correct diagnosis, ultrasound examination, MRI, and computed tomography scans may be useful for further evaluation. Ultrasound examination can reveal hypoechoic fluid within the retrocalcaneal bursa as well as being able to visualize the bony abnormalities associated with Haglund's deformity and calcification within the Achilles tendon.[13,39] MRI provides a more sensitive analysis for assessing the posterior heel.[54] The bony abnormalities of the calcaneus are well visualized on T1-weighted images.[1] An evaluation for bursitis associated with AICT and Haglund's syndrome will show excessive fluid within the retrocalcaneal and superficial bursae, appearing with a low intensity on T1-weighted images and high intensity with T2-weighted imaging.[1,13] When looking at the patient suffering from AICT, MRI may reveal intratendinous and peritendinous edema on T2-weighted images as well as thickening of the insertion with intratendinous areas of increased signal intensity on T1-weighted MRI that is less evident with a T2-weighted image[1,13](**Fig. 6**). MRI can also aid in the decision for the need of a flexor hallucis longus transfer in patients with severe degeneration of the Achilles tendon. Computed tomography imaging of the posterior heel may be useful for preoperative planning, because it will show the exact location and size of the deformities for Haglund's deformity.[39]

Surgical Management

Differentiating the surgical procedure between a Haglund's deformity and AICT is based on the extent of the calcification as well as how much Achilles tendinopathy is present. Typically, in a Haglund's deformity, there is minimal Achilles tendinopathy and the calcification can be accessed without detachment of the Achilles tendon. This procedure is usually performed through a posterior lateral incision along the

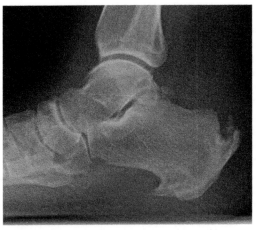

Fig. 4. Lateral radiograph showing the calcification at the attachment site and extending into the Achilles tendon of an AICT.

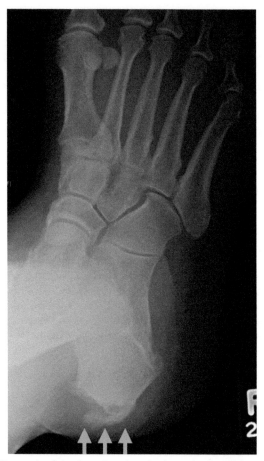

Fig. 5. Oblique radiograph of the foot showing the lateral to medial extension of the calcification of an AICT (*green arrows*).

calcaneus. This incision placement is posterior to the sural nerve and lateral to the Achilles tendon. Occasionally, a small portion of the Achilles tendon along the lateral aspect needs to be reflected to adequately expose the Haglund's protuberance. The superior portion of the calcaneus can also be accessed through this incision to decompress the retrocalcaneal area if needed. Resection of the calcification can be performed using an osteotome and bone rasp. These authors often will resect more bone than just the protuberance anticipating some type of bony regrowth. Once the calcifications have been removed, a bone anchor can be used to not only reapproximate the reflected portion of the Achilles tendon but also allows for a covering over the resected bone, hopefully to minimize regrowth. A single layer closure is performed to try and avoid sural entrapment. Postoperatively, the patient is placed in a nonweightbearing splint in a neutral position for approximately 10 days. At that point, if everything looks good from an incision standpoint, the patient can begin progressive weightbearing in a boot as tolerated. At 4 weeks postoperative, physical therapy is started to advance out of the boot and slowly start to advance activities.

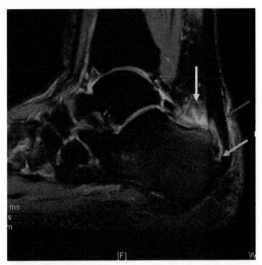

Fig. 6. Sagittal MRI showing the retrocalcaneal bursitis (*yellow arrow*), thickening, and degeneration of the Achilles tendon (*red arrow*) and the calcification of the calcaneus (*green arrow*) with an AICT.

This surgical treatment for AICT is substantially different compared with that for a Haglund's deformity. Because the calcification with this deformity involves a significant portion of the posterior aspect of the Achilles tendon at the attachment and tendinopathy of the Achilles tendon, this procedure normally involves the detachment of the Achilles tendon with a posterior calcaneal ostectomy and repair with reattachment of the Achilles tendon.

The patient is placed in a prone position after a general anesthetic has been administered. A thigh tourniquet is used. The patient is prepped and draped up to the knee. A "step" incision is made along the posterior aspect of the Achilles tendon and calcaneus (**Fig. 7**). The proximal vertical arm of the incision is placed along the medial aspect of the Achilles tendon. The transverse aspect of the incision follows skin tension lines and is placed over the calcification at the attachment site. The distal vertical incision is then extended laterally along the posterior calcaneus. This incision allows for the flaps to be raised without the use of continuous retraction on the skin. Once the Achilles tendon is exposed, a linear incision is made along the distal aspect of the central aspect of the Achilles tendon extending to the insertion site (**Fig. 8**). The medial and lateral halves of the Achilles tendon are detached from the insertion site. At this point, the mucoid degeneration can easily be visualized within the tendon. A sharp 15 blade is used to excise the degeneration, taking care to avoid any over-resection of the Achilles tendon (**Fig. 9**). In patients in whom there is severe mucoid degeneration, a flexor hallucis longus transfer into the calcaneus can be considered. Next, the posterior calcification can be resected at the insertion site and the authors also recommend resection the posterior-superior protuberance off of the calcaneus (**Figs. 10** and **11**). A bone rasp can be used to smooth out any of the rough surfaces. Once the surfaces have been resected and smoothed, the contouring of the calcaneus can be evaluated using intraoperative radiography or fluoroscopy. The goal is to have a smooth contour of the posterior and posterior-superior aspect of the calcaneus (**Fig. 12**). The authors also evaluate the very medial and lateral aspects of the insertion site to make sure there are no sharp ridges that need to be resected.

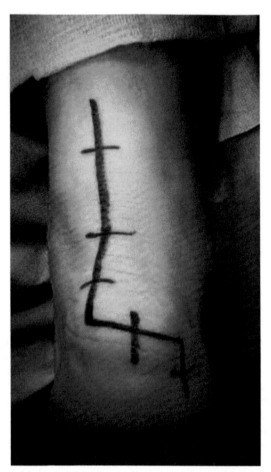

Fig. 7. "Step" incision for AICT.

Once satisfied with the resection, the area is irrigated. Bone wax was then applied to the very superior aspect where the posterior-superior calcaneus was resected. Care is made to avoid any placement of the bone wax at the attachment site. The Achilles tendon is then reattached using the surgeon's preference of a type of bone anchoring system (**Fig. 13**). The foot is held in a plantar flexed position during the reattachment. Once the Achilles tendon has been reattached, the Achilles tendon in is repaired using a running 2-0 nonabsorbable suture. A single layer closure is performed using a combination of absorbable and nonabsorbable sutures or staples.

Postoperatively, the patient is placed in a nonweightbearing plantarflexed splint for approximately 10 days. At 10 days postoperative, the patient is then placed in a plantarflexed removable boot or splint and kept nonweightbearing. The boot or splint can be removed for cleaning of the incision and gentle range of motion exercises of the ankle. At 3 weeks postoperative, if the incision is healed, then the sutures can be removed. The patient is then placed in a weightbearing boot with a 3-layered heel lift. After a week, 1 layer of the heel lift can be removed, and the subsequent layers can be removed on a weekly basis over the next 2 weeks. Range of motion is started as tolerated. Wearing of a weightbearing boot continues until 8 weeks postoperative.

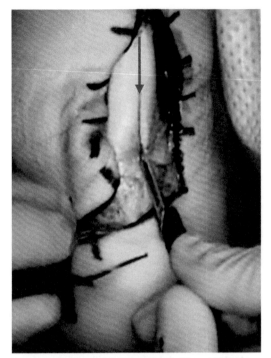

Fig. 8. Longitudinal incision of the Achilles tendon (*red arrow*).

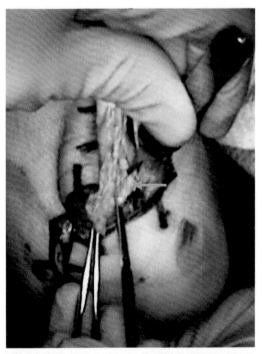

Fig. 9. Resection of the mucoid degeneration of the Achilles tendon (*green arrow*).

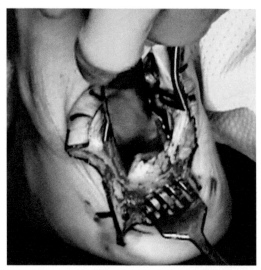

Fig. 10. Resection of the posterior calcification with an osteotome.

At 8 weeks postoperative, the patient can start to wean out of the boot and physical therapy can be started if needed. Patients can expect chronic swelling to the Achilles tendon. It typically takes approximately 9 to 12 months for overall recovery with the posterior calcaneal ostectomy and detachment with repair and reattachment Achilles tendon.

Complications

Complications can occur with either of the procedures for a Haglund's deformity or an AICT. The most common complications that can be seen with a Haglund's deformity

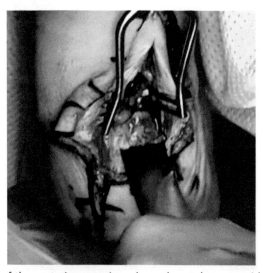

Fig. 11. Resection of the posterior–superior calcaneal protuberance with an osteotome.

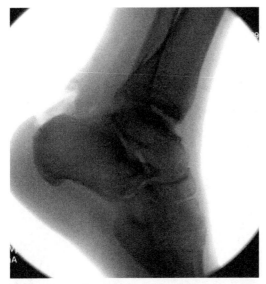

Fig. 12. Intraoperative fluoroscan showing the postresection contouring of the calcaneus.

are irritation or entrapment of the sural nerve. These complications are typically seen owing to the formation of scar tissue along the incision site, entrapping the nerve.

For an AICT, complications can consist of dehiscence of the incision (**Fig. 14**). Care must be taken to make sharp 90° angles at the corners of the incision to help avoid this complication. Recurrence of the calcification at the insertion site is rare, but these authors have seen a number of patients develop heterotopic ossification along the superior aspect of the calcaneus anterior to the Achilles tendon; this complication is typically asymptomatic (**Fig. 15**).

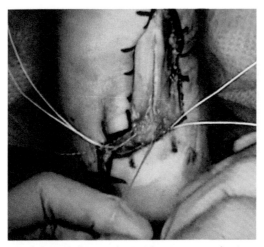

Fig. 13. Reattachment of the Achilles tendon with a suture-anchoring system.

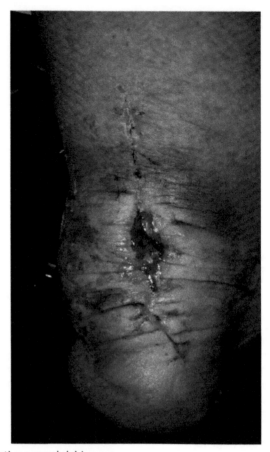

Fig. 14. Postoperative wound dehiscence.

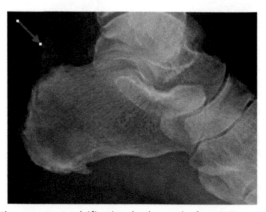

Fig. 15. Postoperative recurrent calcification (*red arrow*) after AICT resection.

CLINICS CARE POINTS

- AICT will cause pain along the entire posterior aspect of the calcaneus that is worse with shoes with high-backed heel counters.
- Achilles tendinosis is common in patients with AICT and uncommon in patients with Haglund's deformity.
- Resection of the AICT involves detachment of the Achilles tendon with reattachment after debridement of the tendinosis.
- Haglund's deformity requires minimal resection of the Achilles tendon.
- Superior heterotopic ossification may occur after resection of the AICT, but is rarely symptomatic.

DISCLOSURE

S.T. Grambart: Partner BESPA Global. No conflicts.

REFERENCES

1. Lawrence DA, Rolen MF, Morshed KA, et al. MRI of heel pain. AJR Am J Roentgenol 2013;200(4):845–55.
2. Michetti ML, Jacobs SA. Calcaneal heel spurs: etiology, treatment, and a new surgical approach. J Foot Surg 1983;22(3):234–9.
3. Vaishya R, Agarwal AK, Azizi AT, et al. Haglund's syndrome: a commonly seen mysterious condition. Cureus 2016;8(10):e820.
4. Barg A, Ludwig T. Surgical strategies for the treatment of insertional Achilles tendinopathy. Foot Ankle Clin 2019;24(3):533–59.
5. Kucuksen S, Karahan AY, Erol K. Haglund syndrome with pump bump. Med Arch 2012;66(6):425–7.
6. Aldridge T. Diagnosing heel pain in adults. Am Fam Physician 2004;70(2):332–8.
7. Gillott E, Ray P. Tuberculosis of the calcaneum masquerading as Haglund's deformity: a rare case and brief literature review. BMJ Case Rep 2013;2013.
8. Kolodziej P, Glisson RR, Nunley JA. Risk of avulsion of the Achilles tendon after partial excision for treatment of insertional tendonitis and Haglund's deformity: a biomechanical study. Foot Ankle Int 1999;20(7):433–7.
9. Krishna Sayana M, Maffulli N. Insertional Achilles tendinopathy. Foot Ankle Clin 2005;10(2):309–20.
10. Le TA, Joseph PM. Common exostectomies of the rearfoot. Clin Podiatr Med Surg 1991;8(3):601–23.
11. Lee JC, Calder JD, Healy JC. Posterior impingement syndromes of the ankle. Semin Musculoskelet Radiol 2008;12(2):154–69.
12. Lopez RG, Jung HG. Achilles tendinosis: treatment options. Clin Orthop Surg 2015;7(1):1–7.
13. Narvaez JA, Narvaez J, Ortega R, et al. Painful heel: MR imaging findings. Radiographics 2000;20(2):333–52.
14. Haglund P. Beitrag zur Klinik der Achillessehne. Zeitschr Orthop Chir 1928;49:49–58.
15. Pavlov H, Heneghan MA, Hersh A, et al. The Haglund syndrome: initial and differential diagnosis. Radiology 1982;144(1):83–8.

16. Pincus AI. Haglund's disease; an analytical review of the syndrome with the report of two surgical cases. J Natl Assoc Chirop 1948;38(8):13–23.

17. Stephens MM. Haglund's deformity and retrocalcaneal bursitis. Orthop Clin North Am 1994;25(1):41–6.

18. Tu P. Heel pain: diagnosis and management. Am Fam Physician 2018;97(2): 86–93.

19. Weinfeld SB. Achilles tendon disorders. Med Clin North Am 2014;98(2):331–8.

20. Johansson KJ, Sarimo JJ, Lempainen LL, et al. Calcific spurs at the insertion of the Achilles tendon: a clinical and histological study. Muscles Ligaments Tendons J 2012;2(4):273–7.

21. Sofka CM, Adler RS, Positano R, et al. Haglund's syndrome: diagnosis and treatment using sonography. HSS J 2006;2(1):27–9.

22. Miller AE, Vogel TA. Haglund's deformity and the Keck and Kelly osteotomy: a retrospective analysis. J Foot Surg 1989;28(1):23–9.

23. Nisbet NW. Tendo Achilles bursitis (winter heel). Br Med J 1954;2(4901):1394–5.

24. Cohen JC. Anatomy and biomechanical aspects of the gastrocsoleus complex. Foot Ankle Clin 2009;14(4):617–26.

25. Sella EJ. Disorders of the Achilles tendon and its insertion. Clin Podiatr Med Surg 2005;22(1):87–99, vii.

26. Chen TM, Rozen WM, Pan WR, et al. The arterial anatomy of the Achilles tendon: anatomical study and clinical implications. Clin Anat 2009;22(3):377–85.

27. Kannus P. Structure of the tendon connective tissue. Scand J Med Sci Sports 2000;10(6):312–20.

28. Alexander RM, Bennet-Clark HC. Storage of elastic strain energy in muscle and other tissues. Nature 1977;265(5590):114–7.

29. Fiamengo SA, Warren RF, Marshall JL, et al. Posterior heel pain associated with a calcaneal step and Achilles tendon calcification. Clin Orthop Relat Res 1982;167: 203–11.

30. Vega MR, Cavolo DJ, Green RM, et al. Haglund's deformity. J Am Podiatry Assoc 1984;74(3):129–35.

31. Carr AJ, Norris SH. The blood supply of the calcaneal tendon. J Bone Joint Surg Br 1989;71(1):100–1.

32. Kvist M. Achilles tendon injuries in athletes. Sports Med 1994;18(3):173–201.

33. Pierre-Jerome C, Moncayo V, Terk MR. MRI of the Achilles tendon: a comprehensive review of the anatomy, biomechanics, and imaging of overuse tendinopathies. Acta Radiol 2010;51(4):438–54.

34. Bottger BA, Schweitzer ME, El-Noueam KI, et al. MR imaging of the normal and abnormal retrocalcaneal bursae. AJR Am J Roentgenol 1998;170(5):1239–41.

35. Reddy SS, Pedowitz DI, Parekh SG, et al. Surgical treatment for chronic disease and disorders of the Achilles tendon. J Am Acad Orthop Surg 2009;17(1):3–14.

36. Heneghan MA, Pavlov H. The Haglund painful heel syndrome. Experimental investigation of cause and therapeutic implications. Clin Orthop Relat Res 1984;187:228–34.

37. Keck SW, Kelly PJ. Bursitis of the posterior part of the heel; evaluation of surgical treatment of eighteen patients. J Bone Joint Surg Am 1965;47:267–73.

38. B B. Development of human synovial bursae. Anat Rec 1934;60:333.

39. van Dijk CN, van Sterkenburg MN, Wiegerinck JI, et al. Terminology for Achilles tendon related disorders. Knee Surg Sports Traumatol Arthrosc 2011;19(5): 835–41.

40. Ortmann FW, McBryde AM. Endoscopic bony and soft-tissue decompression of the retrocalcaneal space for the treatment of Haglund deformity and retrocalcaneal bursitis. Foot Ankle Int 2007;28(2):149–53.
41. Miller BF, Buhr AJ. Pump bumps or knobbly heels. N S Med Bull 1969;48(6): 191–2.
42. Dickinson PHCM, Woodward EP. Tendon Achilles bursitis. J Bone Joint Surg Am 1966;48:77–81.
43. Schneider W, Niehus W, Knahr K. Haglund's syndrome: disappointing results following surgery – a clinical and radiographic analysis. Foot Ankle Int 2000; 21(1):26–30.
44. Lu CC, Cheng YM, Fu YC, et al. Angle analysis of Haglund syndrome and its relationship with osseous variations and Achilles tendon calcification. Foot Ankle Int 2007;28(2):181–5.
45. Reinherz RP, Smith BA, Henning KE. Understanding the pathologic Haglund's deformity. J Foot Surg 1990;29(5):432–5.
46. Ruch JA. Haglund's disease. J Am Podiatry Assoc 1974;64(12):1000–3.
47. Reule CA, Alt WW, Lohrer H, et al. Spatial orientation of the subtalar joint axis is different in subjects with and without Achilles tendon disorders. Br J Sports Med 2011;45(13):1029–34.
48. Resnick D, Feingold ML, Curd J, et al. Calcaneal abnormalities in articular disorders. Rheumatoid arthritis, ankylosing spondylitis, psoriatic arthritis, and Reiter syndrome. Radiology 1977;125(2):355–66.
49. Solan M, Davies M. Management of insertional tendinopathy of the Achilles tendon. Foot Ankle Clin 2007;12(4):597–615, vi.
50. Fowler APJ. Abnormality of the calcaneus as a cause of painful heel. Br J Surg 1945;32:494–8.
51. Singh R, Rohilla R, Siwach RC, et al. Diagnostic significance of radiologic measurements in posterior heel pain. Foot (Edinb) 2008;18(2):91–8.
52. Kang S, Thordarson DB, Charlton TP. Insertional Achilles tendinitis and Haglund's deformity. Foot Ankle Int 2012;33(6):487–91.
53. Chauveaux D, Liet P, Le Huec JC, et al. A new radiologic measurement for the diagnosis of Haglund's deformity. Surg Radiol Anat 1991;13(1):39–44.
54. Kier R. Magnetic resonance imaging of plantar fasciitis and other causes of heel pain. Magn Reson Imaging Clin N Am 1994;2(1):97–107.

Heel Complications

Eric A. Barp, DPM[a,b,]*, Eric R. Reese, DPM[a,b], Nephi E.H. Jones, DPM[a,b],
Zachary J. Bliek, DPM[a,b]

KEYWORDS

- Hypersensitivity reaction • Achilles repair • Suture tape • Nonabsorbable implants
- Suture anchors • Rearfoot complications

KEY POINTS

- Suture anchors can be effective devices to help strengthen surgical fixation when placing the tendon under tension. However, although rare, they also place the patient at increased risk for adverse foreign body reactions.
- Although it is not a common postoperative complication, hypersensitivity reactions can lead to delayed healing, surgical revisions, infections, and amputations, as well as cosmetic and/or psychological issues for the patient.
- It is important to discuss complications from posterior heel surgery with the patient as complications require prolonged immobilization, as well causing a significant financial burden, often requiring additional surgeries and time off work.
- Postoperatively, aggressive postoperative physical therapy, falls, and increasing activity too rapidly will be the biggest risks for tendon re-rupture.

INTRODUCTION

Surgical procedures involving the Achilles tendon are frequently performed by foot and ankle surgeons. It is well published that these procedures carry notable risks inherent to the procedures to include but not exclusive to the following: wound complications, infections, suture reactions, re-rupture, deep vein thrombosis, and neural symptoms.[1–6] Wounds and delayed foreign body reactions are an unfortunate aspect of surgical intervention. As we discuss, the distal aspect of the Achilles tendon is a common location for these types of complications. The lack of subcutaneous tissue and watershed region (2–6 cm proximal to the Achilles tendon insertion) can make these complications ever more prevalent if the surgeon does not take appropriate intraoperative and postoperative cautions to help reduce the risk of occurrence.[4] Currently there is a paucity of information regarding complications of suture anchors; however, in recent years there has been an increase in discussion and published literature. Suture anchors can be effective devices to help strengthen surgical fixation when placing the tendon under tension. However, although rare, they also place the

[a] The Iowa Clinic, 5950 University Avenue West, Des Moines, IA 50266, USA; [b] Unitypoint Health - Iowa Methodist Medical Center, 1415 Woodland Avenue, Des Moines, IA 50309, USA
* Corresponding author. 5950 University Avenue West, Des Moines, IA 50266.
E-mail address: ebarp@iowaclinic.com

Clin Podiatr Med Surg 38 (2021) 183–191
https://doi.org/10.1016/j.cpm.2020.12.004
0891-8422/21/© 2020 Elsevier Inc. All rights reserved.

podiatric.theclinics.com

patient at increased risk for adverse foreign body reactions. It is important to discuss all these complications, as they require prolonged immobilization, as well as significant financial burden often requiring additional surgeries and time off work.

MANAGEMENT OF SPECIFIC COMPLICATIONS
Overcorrection

Proper intraoperative assessment is necessary to ensure that lengthening will allow the ankle to dorsiflex to neutral position. The Achilles tendon is oftentimes advanced proximally to relieve some of the insertional strain.[7] If this is over advanced or combined with a lengthening, weakness of the triceps surae can ensue and potentially result in a calcaneal gait, although to date we do not believe this has been reported in the literature. Calcaneal gait is defined as increased ankle dorsiflexion during the midstance phase, which in turn places the heel under a longer weight-bearing phase. In a healthy adult with normal biomechanics, the calcaneal gait will be temporary and should resolve as strength is increased during the postoperative phase. If a patient develops pain due to increased heel weight bearing, conservative therapies such as physical therapy to strengthen the posterior muscle group and orthotics with padded heel cup have been anecdotally beneficial. Gastrocnemius recessions are not typically done in adjunct to these therapies, as we feel that this could lead to overcorrection and further complications.

Patients may also experience continued postoperative pain from overaggressive resection of the insertional spur or retrocalcaneal exostosis, as well as bone resorption around anchors used to reattach the Achilles tendon. This typically can be resolved with postoperative physical therapy and nonsteroidal anti-inflammatory drugs (NSAIDS).

Achilles Tendinosis/Rupture

Rupture of the Achilles tendon after surgical correction of insertional pathology is rare.[8] We routinely obtain MRIs of our patients with both posterior heel and Achilles pathology to ensure they are adequately treated with conservative and surgical measures. If tendon pathology is seen in the watershed zone (2–6 cm proximal to the Achilles tendon insertion), we recommend resection of all pathologic tendon and lengthening the postoperative recovery period to allow complete healing.[9] With respect to rupture following repair with suture anchors, the tendon or suture will tear before anchor fixation fails.[10,11] This will most commonly occur at the point where the tendon twists, an anatomic location that is at risk for rupture.[12] Postoperatively, aggressive postoperative physical therapy, falls, and increasing activity too rapidly will be the biggest risks for tendon rupture. If a rupture does occur postoperatively, surgical revision is warranted.

Infections and Delayed Wound Healing

Infections in the posterior heel area need to be treated aggressively because of the lack of subcutaneous tissue interface between the tendon and skin. We recommend treating with oral antibiotics if possible and local wound care. If infection persists, worsens, or deepens, all suture material should be removed, as it can serve as a nidus for deeper infections. Primary closure should be considered after debridement; however, delayed primary closure may be necessary due to soft tissue defects. Highlander and Greenhagen[5] undertook a systematic review looking at complication rates between posterior midline and posterior medial incisions and the cumulative data found wound complication rates of 7.0% of patients undergoing a posterior midline incision and 8.3% of patients who have posterior medial incisions. The complications accounted for skin edge necrosis, delayed healing, and painful/hypertrophic scars. To avoid complications, we recommend several intraoperative protocols. The skin incision placement should follow angiosome intersection either midline or slightly lateral. A medially deviated incision should be avoided. Maintain full-thickness skin flaps and avoid overdissection of tissue layers between skin and bone. Too much dissection will disrupt the delicate vascular network. Separation of layers can also lead to seroma formation. Careful skin handling intraoperatively by using self-retaining retractors or the no-touch suturing technique should be used. Both will minimize human error of overaggressive retraction. The most commonly encountered wound-healing complication is dehiscence at the distal incision at the transition of supple skin to more glabrous skin.[13–18] Aggressive wound therapy will typically warrant success. We typically start with our in-office wound care specialist and close follow–up. Considerations should be made for secondary wound closure, plastic surgery, or vascular surgery consultation if the wound does not respond appropriately.

Deep Vein Thrombosis

We routinely prescribe deep venous thrombosis (DVT) prophylactic medication to patients undergoing posterior heel surgery. Postoperatively, the patient is immobilized in a posterior splint to eliminate ankle motion and hold the ankle in neutral position. The incidence of DVT occurrence after posterior heel surgery has been poorly reported, and prophylaxis guidelines do not recommend prophylaxis for routine foot and ankle surgery.[19] An observational study in 2013 found that without thromboprophylaxis, the highest incidence of DVT in foot and ankle surgery occurred after repair of Achilles tendon ruptures.[20] Given the morbidity, potential long-term complications, and potential fatal outcomes of a progressive DVT to pulmonary embolism, we have elected to provide thromboprophylaxis to our patients until they can begin physical therapy.

Neural Symptoms

The sural nerve provides branches to the posterior calcaneus that lie in close proximity to the incision. Excessive retraction, lateral dissection, and posterior lateral ankle incisions can result in neurologic symptoms. Resolution is patient dependent. Care should be taken when dissecting in these areas to prevent permanent nerve damage. With a lateral approach, altered sensation postoperatively has been reported as high as 40%.[21] Because the sural nerve and its branches are responsible for sensory and not motor functions, injury here has been well tolerated by individuals. Many reported cases have gone on to resolve spontaneously over time. In the event that neurosensory alteration results in pain, we recommend treating with desensitization therapy, massaging the skin, and corticosteroid injections.

Hypersensitivity Reactions

Hypersensitivity reactions from implantable materials, including absorbable and nonabsorbable suture material, although not a common postoperative complication, when it does occur can lead to chronic pain, delayed healing, surgical revisions, infections, and amputations, as well as cosmetic and/or psychological issues for the patient.

In 1963, Gell and Coombs[22] published their classifications on allergic (hypersensitivity) reactions, categorizing them into 4 subtypes based on the type of immune response and the mechanism for cell and tissue damage.[23] The subtypes include Type I, immediate or immunoglobulin (Ig)E mediated; Type II, cytotoxic or IgG/IgM mediated; Type III, IgG/IgM complex mediated; and Type IV, delayed hypersensitivity or T-cell mediated. Since its publication in 1963, numerous articles, including Uzzaman and Cho,[23] have improved on the Gell and Coombs classification.[22] For the intent of this article, we shall not delve deeper into the changes to the classification but concentrate on a brief overview of Type IV allergic (hypersensitivity) reaction.

Type IV or delayed hypersensitivity reaction is mediated by CD4+ T-helper cells (Th1-type response). Tissue injury is primarily caused by lysosomal enzymes, reactive oxygen intermediates, nitric oxide, and proinflammatory cytokines that are secreted by activated macrophages. This secretion of cytokines and growth factors often leads to fibrosis of the tissue and the formation of granulomatous reaction.[23] Tissue injury/damage, as seen with surgical incisions and disruption of tissue layers during dissection, can stimulate the release of proinflammatory cytokines stimulating the activation of macrophages. Once activated, macrophages use the process of phagocytosis to engulf particles and then digest them. Catelas and colleagues[24] researched cell-mediated responses to both ceramic and polyethylene particles and found that particles small enough to undergo phagocytosis by macrophages (<7 μm) were able to incite a cell-mediated inflammatory response. They also concluded that macrophage response to polyethylene debris was dependent on both the size and concentration. With this knowledge, the foot and ankle surgeon should always be concerned with the type, size, and amount of implantable suture material used to reduce the risk of a hypersensitivity or granulomatous-type reaction.[25] If a hypersensitivity reaction does occur and any conservative measures fail, we recommend removal of the offending sutures and anchors as well as obtaining intraoperative soft tissue and bone cultures to ensure no other pathologic process is present.

Fiberwire/Suture Tape

With drastic change in most postoperative protocols leaning toward early weight bearing and mobilization in orthopedic surgery the use of suture tape by the orthopedic community has become appealing due to the properties it possesses. More specifically, FiberWire consists of a core that is multithreaded polyethylene with a braided jacket consisting of polyester.[26] These components give FiberWire excellent strength, resistance to tension, and knot-tying ability. There are other high-tensile sutures that consist of polyethylene and polyester but FiberWire is unique in that it has an outer silicone coating. Ticron is the only other high-tensile suture in the United States that has an outer silicone coating.[27]

Suture tape is appealing when faced with an Achilles tendon repair due to the high tensile and strength properties it possesses. The use of this suture will allow you to maintain tendon apposition while using early weight bearing and mobilization. As reported by the literature, FiberWire seems to be common for this repair. Recent literature on complications associated with FiberWire may suggest otherwise.

FiberWire has been shown to cause foreign body reactions resulting in an increase in the number of reoperations. Recent literature as shown complications with the use of tightropes can lead to osteolysis and stitch abscess.[28] Willmott and colleagues[29] performed a retrospective study on 6 patients who had treatment of ankle diastasis with the use of a tightrope. Two (33%) of the 6 patients had to have the tightrope removed because of soft tissue irritation. Histopathologic analysis in one patient confirmed a reaction to foreign body.[29] Ollivere and colleagues[25] reported a case on a minimally invasive Achilles tendon repair with the use of Ethibond and FiberWire. The patient returned to the clinic at 8 months with a swollen Achilles tendon. Foreign body reaction to FiberWire was confirmed with ultrasound and histopathological analysis of tissue surrounding the suture. This hypersensitivity reaction caused a 5-cm cross-sectional area of degenerate tendon that had to be removed. The patient was treated with a flexor hallucis longus transfer. The patient had no complications following the revision at 6 months postoperation but was unable to perform a single heel rise.

Mack and colleagues[27] reported a granulomatous reaction in their case series of 178 patients where FiberWire was used for myodesis in traumatic lower extremity amputations. There were 5 amputations that developed sinus tracts due to a foreign body reaction from previously healed incisions. Mack and colleagues[27] took a unique approach to the study with the use of scanning electron microscopy with energy dispersive x-ray analysis. They used this imaging to show that the gel material found within the giant cells was in fact silicone. They concluded that because the hypersensitivity reaction only occurred in 3% (5/178) of the patients that the silicone coating on the suture must be only a part of the problem. When looking at the etiology of the reaction, there are other components that could be playing a role, such as suture prominence combined with repetitive motion and shear, which could be linked to the inflammatory process within the tissue surrounding the suture.[27]

Hypersensitivity Reaction: Case Reports

Patient 1
A 45-year-old healthy male firefighter was seen 4 weeks status post insertional calcific spur resection after tripping on stairs while not wearing his CAM boot. MRI confirmed an acute midsubstance Achilles tendon rupture. The Achilles rupture was surgically repaired with suture tape using a Krackow stitch. The tail ends were passed subcutaneously to 2 small stab incisions on the posterior heel and anchored into the posterior aspect of the calcaneus for additional support. Approximately 28 weeks postoperatively, he began to experience new-onset pain and swelling with activity. Repeat MRI indicated a re-rupture of the right Achilles tendon. He was placed in a below-knee cast. After 2 to 3 weeks, he developed increased tightness in the right ankle and the cast was removed. A repeat MRI was performed that demonstrated increased uptake to the anchor and nonabsorbable suture. He underwent removal of the remaining suture tape and anchors. The area was flushed with normal saline with bacitracin, and calcaneal bone cultures were taken for microbiology and pathology. Cultures were negative and pathology was unremarkable. The postoperative course was uneventful, with complete healing at 4 weeks (**Figs. 1** and **2**).

Patient 2
A 65-year-old healthy man with past history positive only for previous knee surgery and rotator cuff repair was seen after falling off a ladder landing on his left foot. He was diagnosed with an acute Achilles tendon rupture and underwent surgical repair of his left Achilles tendon. A suture tape was used to secure the tendon edges with a Krackow suture technique and the tails were passed percutaneously, then secured into the posterior aspect of the calcaneus with two 4.7-mm bone anchors. At postoperative week 45, he returned to the clinic with increased redness and pain, along with an open wound. An MRI was performed demonstrating a foreign body reaction to retained bone anchors and embedded suture material. During surgical removal of the suture tape and bone anchors, 2 bone specimens were taken from the calcaneus for culture and pathology to rule out osteomyelitis. The results of the microbiology cultures were negative for bacteria, and pathology was negative for osteomyelitis. The patient had complete resolution at 3 weeks (**Fig. 3**).

DISCUSSION

Surgical procedures are unfortunately not without risk of associated complications. Some foot and ankle procedures have much higher risks for postoperative

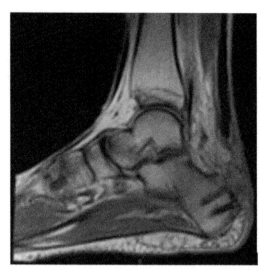

Fig. 1. T1 image 4 weeks status post insertional calcific spur resection.

complications than others, as we know through experience, diligent research, and available published literature. It is important to discuss all potential complications for the surgical procedure, as they often require prolonged immobilization, which can lead to a significant financial burden through extended time off work and additional surgeries. Preoperative patient education on potential postoperative complications is paramount to help ease some of the emotional and mental burden that can accrue for both the patient and surgeon. It can also help prevent noncompliance. It is imperative that the foot and ankle surgeon be well aware of the most frequent complications associated with the procedures being performed. A thorough history and

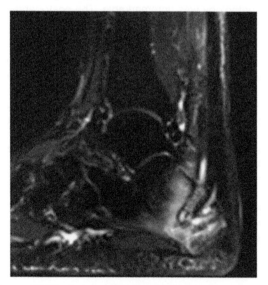

Fig. 2. T2 image demonstrating increased uptake in the suture anchor and nonabsorbable suture tape.

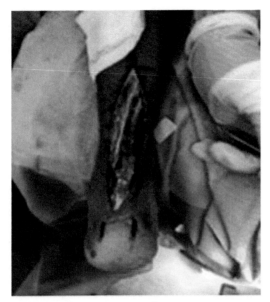

Fig. 3. Repair of Achilles tendon with suture anchors.

physical examination protects the surgeon and patient from many avoidable complications. In many cases, these patients may require treatment from other specialties to ensure that they are optimized for healing before proceeding with elective surgical procedures. Again, patient education should not be minimized. This is an important part of the process, allowing the patient to become his or her own advocate. Informing the patient about how their decisions affect the potential outcome of their surgical procedures has been shown to be effective in minimizing noncompliance.[30]

CLINICS CARE POINTS

Technique Pearls and Pitfalls to Avoid Complications
- Incision placement and tissue handling are some of the basic principles to help avoid postoperative complications. Knowing and understanding the angiosomes to the posterior heel will help guide incision placement and avoid vascular embarrassment. There are 2 main angiosomes to consider on the posterior heel. These lay both medial and lateral to the Achilles tendon. Incisions are best made midline over the Achilles tendon, as this central area divides the 2 angiosomes. In 2006, Attinger and colleagues[4] set forth 4 principles when considering incision placement. These are as follows: (1) incision must provide adequate exposure for the planned procedure, (2) there must be adequate blood supply on either side of the incision for optimal healing, (3) incision should spare sensory and motor nerves, and (4) incision should not be perpendicular to a joint. With any incision at an increased risk for nonhealing, a "no-touch" technique should be utilized.
- Another basic principle to help avoid postoperative complications is as simple as positioning. Generally, for posterior heel surgery, the patient should be placed in a prone position to allow for easy and adequate exposure for the procedure to be performed. When prone, the patient's foot should hang over the end of the table on a pillow to allow for neutral plantar flexion of the foot by elevating the leg and flexing the knee to remove tension on the Achilles tendon while allowing ease of exposure to the calcaneal tuberosity. This also will allow for minimal tissue handling and reduce soft tissue trauma.

- Thigh tourniquets should be used over the use of a calf tourniquet for any posterior heel surgery. A calf tourniquet will compress and restrict motion within the gastro soleus complex. A thigh tourniquet will allow for full range of motion of the ankle during the posterior heel surgery. A surgeon may opt to not use a tourniquet but this may lead to longer operative times and increased anesthesia requirements for the patient.
- General anesthesia is absolutely necessary for optimal surgical outcomes with posterior heel procedures. Complete paralysis is necessary throughout the procedure for assessing range of motion and during the repair. General anesthesia also will prevent inadvertent movements by the patient due to pain/stimulation of the procedure and the thigh tourniquet.
- Although uncommon, DVT can have potentially fatal outcomes. Postoperatively, the patient is immobilized in a posterior splint to eliminate ankle motion and hold correction with the ankle in neutral position. DVT prophylaxis is generally not recommended in routine foot and ankle surgery; however, an observational study in 2013 by Lapidus and colleagues[20] found that without DVT prophylaxis, the highest incidence of DVT in foot and ankle surgery occurred after repair of Achilles tendon ruptures. The authors routinely prescribe DVT prophylactic medications to patients undergoing posterior heel surgery because of the potential long-term complications or fatal outcomes of a potential DVT.

DISCLOSURE

The authors have nothing to disclose.

REFERENCES

1. Dalton GP, Wapner KL, Hecht PJ. Complications of Achilles and posterior tibial tendon surgeries. Clin Orthop Relat Res 2001;Oct(391):133–9.
2. Nunley JA, Ruskin G, Horst F. Long term clinical outcomes following the central incision technique for insertional Achilles tendinopathy. Foot Ankle Int 2011; 32(9):850–5.
3. Van Dijk CN, Van Sterkenburg MN, Wiegerinck JI, et al. Terminology for Achilles tendon related disorders. Knee Surg Sports Traumatol Arthrosc 2011;19(5):835–41.
4. Attinger CE, Evans KK, Bulan E, et al. Angiosomes of the foot and ankle and clinical implications for limb salvage, reconstruction, incisions, and revascularization. Plast Reconstr Surg 2006;117(7S):261S–93S.
5. Highlander P, Greenhagen RM. Wound complications with posterior midline and posterior medial leg incisions a systematic review. Foot Ankle Spec 2011;4(6): 361–9.
6. Kelikian AS, Sarrafian SK, editors. Sarrafian's anatomy of the foot and ankle: descriptive, topographic, functional. Philadelphia: Lippincott Williams & Wilkins; 2011.
7. Boffeli TJ, Peterson MC. The Keck and Kelly wedge calcaneal osteotomy for Haglund's deformity: a technique for reproducible results. J Foot Ankle Surg 2012; 51(3):398–401.
8. Kolodziej P, Glisson RR, Nunley JA. Risk of avulson of the Achilles tendon after partial excision for treatment of insertional tendonitis and Haglunds deformity: a biomechanical study. Foot Ankle Int 1999;20(7):433–7.
9. Beitzel K, Mazzocca AD, Obopilwe E, et al. Biomechanical properties of double and single row suture anchor repair for surgical treatment of insertional Achilles tendinopathy. Am J Sports Med 2013;41(7):1642–8.
10. Pilson H, Brown P, Stitzel J, et al. Single row versus double row repair of distal Achilles tendon: a biomechanical comparison. J Foot Ankle Surg 2012;51(6):762–6.
11. Maffuli N, Testa V, Capsso G, et al. Calcific insertional Achilles tendinopathy reattachment with bone anchors. Am J Sports Med 2004;32(1):174–82.

12. Witt BL, Hyer CF. Achilles tendon reattachment after surgical treatment of insertional tendinosis using the suture bridge technique: a case series. J Foot Ankle Surg 2012;51(4):487–93.
13. Roche AJ, Calder JDF. Achilles tendinopathy: a review of the current concepts of treatment. Bone Joint J 2013;95-B:1299–307.
14. Paavola M, Kannus P, Orava S, et al. Surgical treatment for chronic Achilles tendinopathy: a prospective seven month follow up study. Br J Sports Med 2002; 36(3):178–82.
15. Calder JDF, Saxby TS. Surgical treatment of insertional Achilles tendinosis. Foot Ankle Int 2003;24(2):119–21.
16. McGarvey WC, Palumbo RC, Baxter DE, et al. Insertional Achilles tendinosis: surgical treatment through a central tendon splitting approach. Foot Ankle Int 2002; 23(1):19–25.
17. Den Hartog BD. Insertional Achilles tendinosis: pathogenesis and treatment. Foot Ankle Clin 2009;14(4):639–50.
18. Murphy GA. Surgical treatment of non insertional Achilles tendinitis. Foot Ankle Clin 2009;14(4):651–61.
19. Falck-Ytter Y, Francis CW, Johanson NA, et al. Prevention of VTE in orthopedic surgery patients: antithrombotic therapy and prevention of thrombosis: American College of Chest Physicians evidence based clinical practice guidelines. Chest J 2012;141(2_suppl):e278S–325S.
20. Lapidus LJ, Ponzer S, Pettersson H, et al. Symptomatic venous thromboembolism and mortality in orthopaedic surgery and observational study of 45,968 consecutive procedures. BMC Musculoskelet Disord 2013;14(1):177.
21. Yodlowski ML, Scheller AD, Minos L. Surgical treatment of Achilles tendinitis by decompression of the retrocalcaneal bursa and the superior calcaneal tuberosity. Am J Sports Med 2002;30(3):318–21.
22. Gell PGH, Coombs RRA. The classification of allergic reactions underlying disease. In: Coombs RRA, Gell PGH, editors. Clinical aspects of immunology. Blackwell Science; 1963.
23. Uzzaman A, Cho S. Classifications of hypersensitivity reactions. Allergy Asthma Proc 2012;33(Supplement 1):S96–9, 4.
24. Catelas I, Petit A, Marchand R, et al. Cytotoxicity and macrophage cytokine release induced by ceramic and polyethylene particles in vitro. J Bone Joint Surg Br 1999;81(3):516–21.
25. Ollivere BJ, Bosman HA, Bearcroft PWP, et al. Foreign body granulomatous reaction associated with polyethelene 'Fiberwire®' suture material used in Achilles tendon repair. JFAS 2014;20:e27–9.
26. Arthrex, Inc.. FiberWire® braided composite suture product brochure. Naples (FL): Arthrex, Inc.; 2005.
27. Mack AW, Freedman BA, Shawen B, et al. Wound complications following the use of fiberwire in lower-extremity traumatic amputations. J Bone Joint Surg Am 2009; 91(3):680–5.
28. Storey P, Gadd RJ, Blundell C, et al. Complications of suture button ankle syndesmosis stabilization with modifications of surgical technique. Foot Ankle Int 2012; 33(9):717–21.
29. Willmott HS, Singh B, David LA. Outcome and complications of treatment of ankle diastasis with tightrope fixation. Injury 2009;40:1204–6.
30. Barp E, Erickson J. Complications of tendon surgery in the foot and ankle. Clin Podiatric Med Surg 2016;33(1):163–75.

Plantar Fasciitis/Fasciosis

Travis Motley, DPM, MS

KEYWORDS

- Plantar fasciitis • Plantar fasciosis • Plantar heel pain

KEY POINTS

- Most of the patients improve with conservative modalities.
- Multiple conservative modalities are successful in the treatment of plantar fasciitis.
- Patients with acute plantar fasciitis generally respond more rapidly and more predictably than patients with chronic plantar fasciitis.
- Patients that undergo endoscopic plantar fasciotomy usually return to activity more promptly than patients that undergo open plantar fasciotomy.

INTRODUCTION

The plantar fascia (or aponeurosis) is described as dense connective tissue, primarily fibrocytes that serves as a link between the origin on the plantar medial tubercle of the calcaneus and the forefoot. The proximal attachment to the calcaneus is fibrocartilaginous.[1] The plantar fascia is divided into the medial, lateral, and central bands.[2] The medial and lateral bands are variable.[3,4] The central band is triangular, varies in width, and divides into 5 longitudinal bands at the midmetatarsal level. These bands subsequently divide at the metatarsal head level into deep and superficial tracts.[5] The thicker central portion adjacent to the 2 thinner lateral and medial fascial bands functions to support the arch of the foot and transmits forces during the gait cycle.[6] Immunohistochemical investigations have shown that almost all of the plantar fascia are type I collagen with free and encapsulated nerve endings.[7,8]

Terminology regarding fasciitis has been appropriately divided into fasciitis (inflammation) and fasciosis (degeneration), which usually follows. Differentiating between fasciitis and fasciosis is really more of a histologic finding. Both are accurate terms with fasciitis better describing acute pain with inflammation and fasciosis describing more chronic, noninflammatory pain. Both terms can be correct depending on the stage of the disease. Fasciitis is commonly used and will be used to describe both pathologies. Plantar fasciitis is a common presentation to the foot and ankle surgeons; several investigators estimate it accounts for about 1 million outpatient visits per year.[9–14] Traditionally, plantar fasciitis is classified as an overuse injury where

Podiatric Surgical Residency, John Peter Smith Hospital, Acclaim Physician Group, 1500 S. Main Street, 3rd Floor OPC Building, Fort Worth, TX 76104, USA
E-mail address: tmotley@jpshealth.org

Clin Podiatr Med Surg 38 (2021) 193–200
https://doi.org/10.1016/j.cpm.2020.12.005
0891-8422/21/© 2021 Elsevier Inc. All rights reserved.

podiatric.theclinics.com

repetitive microtrauma occur to the plantar fascia more frequently than its ability to heal.[13,15] Continuous tension and microtears can lead to a diastasis between the proximal plantar fascia and the calcaneus, which can become filled with new reactive bone and form a spur.[16] Many prior studies have evaluated the increased risk of plantar fasciitis with increased body mass index (>30 kg/m^2), poor choice in shoe gear, increasing activity, and poor activity surfaces.[10,17] Incidence of plantar fasciitis increases between 40 and 60 years of age and is more common in active individuals.[12,18–20] Symptoms resolve in more than 80% of patients with nonoperative treatment.[21] It has been estimated that 10% of patients will not improve with conservative care in the acute phase.[22]

Plantar calcaneal spurs have been reported in those with and without plantar fasciitis.[9] Although often associated with plantar fasciitis, prior anatomic studies have shown that the plantar calcaneal spurs have been shown to originate from the intrinsic muscle attachments rather than the plantar fascia.[23,24] Calcaneal spurs have been classified based on those that occur superior to the plantar fascia than those that are within the plantar fascia. Spurs occurring within the plantar fascia in patients with plantar fasciitis were found to have more inflammation on MRI and histologic studies than those spurs arising superior to the plantar fascia.[25]

DIAGNOSIS

The most common complaint of plantar fascial pain is pain first step out of bed in the morning that tends to decrease with continued activity. Pain recurs when activity resumes after a period of rest. Occasionally, patients will complain of pain throughout the day and with increased activity and pain on direct pressure of the plantar medial tubercle of the calcaneus. Mild edema may be present. Bruising in the area is not seen with plantar fasciitis unless there is an associated rupture or avulsion.

A consensus statement by the American College of Foot and Ankle Surgeons has previously recommended that diagnosis of nontraumatic plantar fasciitis is achieved with appropriate history, physical, and clinical examination. Furthermore, routine radiographs, ultrasonography, or advanced imaging is not necessary.[26] Radiographs and advanced imaging are reserved when there is failure of conservative modalities or in patients who are poor historians. Ankle equinus, more specifically gastrocnemius equinus,[27] is commonly associated with plantar fasciitis although some studies have shown no difference in ankle dorsiflexion from control groups.[28]

TREATMENT

Conservative treatment is the mainstay with plantar fasciitis. There are different outcomes between acute and chronic plantar fasciitis. Although specific rule exist, acute plantar fasciitis is described in studies as less than 8 weeks duration, whereas chronic plantar fasciitis is described as pain for greater than 3 months. The purpose of the differentiation from chronic to acute is that patients presenting with more recent onset of their plantar fascial pain have a quicker and more predictable response to conservative treatment compared with those patients presenting with long-duration plantar fascial pain. Although this division of acute and chronic pain leaves some patients in the middle as far as classification of their presentation, the treatment often remains the same although the duration of treatment and advancing to surgical options is more likely in the patient with chronic plantar fascial pain. Conservative treatment options include strapping, stretching, nonsteroidal antiinflammatory drugs (NSAIDs), corticosteroid injections, platelet-rich plasma injections, autologous whole blood injections, prefabricated orthotics, custom orthotics, night splints, electrotherapy, needling, prolotherapy (proliferation therapy), and extracorporeal shock wave therapy to name a few.

Gastrosoleal and plantar fascial–specific stretching exercises have shown to be effective in reducing pain. In prospective randomized trials by DiGiovanni and colleagues,[29,30] plantar fascial–specific stretching exercises demonstrated continued pain relief greater than gastrosoleal stretches alone in combination with prefabricated inserts and NSAIDs. Combining prefabricated inserts with stretching protocols has been shown to provide better pain relief than with stretching and custom foot orthoses.[20]

Corticosteroid injections decrease inflammation[21] with the goal of breaking the inflammatory cycle and reducing pain. Studies evaluating the effectiveness of corticosteroid injections vary in the number of injections, the frequency of injections (once vs weekly), the site of injection (medial vs plantar), and the technique of injection (simple injection vs a peppering technique of multiple passes of the needle through the area of maximal tenderness). For this reason, any meta-analysis of corticosteroid injection effectiveness must be reviewed critically.

Many studies have demonstrated the effectiveness of corticosteroid injection in comparison to other conservative modalities such as platelet-rich plasma, which has been used for plantar fasciitis treatment based on prior studies due to its ability to promote tissue regeneration.[31,32] Case reports demonstrate decrease in pain with short-term (3 months)[33] and longer-term follow-up (1 year).[34] A single injection of corticosteroid was compared with a single platelet-rich plasma injection and showed similar results in patients with chronic plantar fasciitis.[35] A randomized controlled trial compared corticosteroid injection with dry needling of the plantar fascia with similar results at 3 weeks and dry needling with better pain relief at 6 months without other conservative modalities such as NSAIDs and stretching.[36] Another randomized controlled trial in patients with chronic plantar fasciitis found that platelet-rich plasma injection is better than corticosteroid injection or placebo. All patients also used NSAIDs and stretching protocols. At 18-month follow-up, all groups significantly improved from baseline, where the corticosteroid group had better pain relief in short-term, and the platelet-rich plasma group had better long-term pain relief.[37] In a randomized controlled trial of patients with chronic plantar fasciitis who received single injections of corticosteroid and autologous whole blood, the corticosteroid group had a more rapid decrease in pain in the short term, but by 6 months there were no significant difference between groups.[38] In another randomized controlled trial that evaluated plantar fasciitis in obese patients, those receiving 3 weekly injections of corticosteroid had better pain reduction and improved function compared with those receiving platelet-rich plasma injections.[39] Large meta-analysis of prospective comparative studies in chronic plantar fasciitis that compared platelet-rich plasma with corticosteroids showed that the platelet-rich plasma injection group had a favorable functional outcome and pain control at intermediate and long-term follow-up in comparison to corticosteroid injection.[40]

Extracorporeal shock wave therapy uses single-pulse acoustic waves to a specific site and has been described to treat plantar fasciitis. The mechanism is not fully defined but may involve stimulation of healing with neovascularization, direct suppressive effects on nociceptors, and might provoke fibroblast proliferation to enhance healing.[41,42] Rompe and colleagues[43] evaluated extracorporeal shock-wave therapy in a randomized controlled trial of patients with chronic plantar fasciitis with evaluation at 6 months and at 5 years. Three applications of 1000 impulses of low energy was compared with 3 applications of 10 impulses of low-energy shock waves. No concomitant treatment such as stretching, inserts, or NSAIDs was used. The group with 1000 impulses had better pain reduction at 6 months. Patients with 10 impulses were more likely to have surgical intervention due to continued pain. A randomized controlled trial in patients with chronic plantar fasciitis who had failed prior treatment with NSAIDs, night splints, and heel cups evaluated extracoporeal shock wave therapy, platelet-rich plasma injection, corticosteroid injection, and prolotherapy. All treatments were once a week for 3 weeks. At a 36-month follow-up, no significant difference was found between treatment groups.[44] In contrast, another study[45] found in acute plantar fascial pain that a single corticosteroid injection was superior to 3 weekly extracorporeal shock wave applications.

Surgical treatment of plantar fasciitis is reserved for the small percentage that fail conservative modalities. Both open and endoscopic procedures for division of the plantar fascia have been described. Previous reports also include limited division of the gastrocnemius to address concomitant gastrocnemius equinus. Monteagudo and colleagues[46] reported that only 60% of patients who underwent open plantar fasciotomy for chronic plantar fascial pain reported satisfactory results and required 10 weeks to return to work, whereas 95% of those who underwent proximal medial gastrocnemius release reported satisfactory results in and were able to return to work in 3 weeks. Barrett and Day[47] first described the endoscopic plantar fasciotomy technique. Early reports describe the importance of only partial proximal fasciotomy to prevent destabilization of the lateral or medial columns.[48] This partial fasciotomy is described correctly as the medial half of the central band of the plantar fascia. A retrospective evaluation of endoscopic to open plantar fasciotomy for chronic plantar fasciitis showed patients who underwent the endoscopic procedure went back to work, on average, 55 days sooner than those patients underwent open fasciotomy with heel spur resection.[49] Other studies have described endoscopic plantar fasciotomy procedure superior to open procedure in less postoperative pain, quicker return to work, and lower complications rates.[48,50] Other endoscopic techniques for debridement of the plantar fascia or fasciotomy have been described.[51,52]

DISCUSSION

Diagnosis and correct treatment of plantar fasciitis relies on history and clinical examination. More advanced radiographic modalities are reserved for patients with persistent pain or those patients with an uncertain clinical examination. Patients with acute plantar fasciitis are more likely to have a successful outcome than those with a delayed presentation and chronic pain.[53,54] Patients with chronic plantar fascial pain may have an unpredictable response to any form of treatment.[55] Prior studies have found that 90% of patients with plantar fasciitis improve with conservative treatment options at an average of 8 to 10 months from onset of symptoms.[56,57] Long-term follow-up studies may not have significant clinical value because plantar fasciitis is commonly accepted as a self-limiting process. For example, what is the value of a 5-year follow-up when 80% to 90% of patients have decreased pain with or without treatment within that time frame?

Multiple conservative treatment options have been described and compared with control groups, sham treatments, or one or more treatment groups. These options include gastrosoleal and plantar fascial–specific stretching exercises, NSAIDs, corticosteroid injections, oral steroids, taping or strapping, prefabricated or custom orthoses, autologous whole blood injections, platelet-rich plasma injections, dry needling techniques, and others. In short, almost all conservative modalities decrease pain, and the differences may be statistically significant but may not demonstrate any significant clinical result. Most outcomes are measured in visual pain scores or function indices. Although these are validated outcome measures, patients have different pain tolerances and different expectations with pain relief, so those results have to be taken in context. The most frequent comparison of a treatment modality for plantar fasciitis is to corticosteroid injection, which suggests that corticosteroid injection is a common practice probably due to the low cost and low risk of any complications. Although corticosteroid injections are commonly used for plantar fasciitis, there is no consensus on the frequency, interval, or technique of injection.

It is important to recognize the realm of conservative treatment options that are available to the foot and ankle specialist. It is important to consider the cost associated with care. Some of the conservative options have specific cost-of-care benefits such as the cost difference between prefabricated versus custom orthotics and platelet-rich plasma versus corticosteroid injections. Not all conservative treatment options work for all patients. If one particular treatment does not offer relief, continue to other options considering the different expectations in acute and chronic plantar fascial pain. For example, many studies show superiority of corticosteroid injections to extracorporeal shock wave therapy in the acute phase. It seems that in the acute phase the features of a failed healing response are not yet present and the healing process induced by extracorporeal shock wave therapy would not play a role in the acute phase.[45] Although there are many randomized controlled trials for plantar fasciitis, it seems that the mainstay of treatment remains conservative care.

CLINICS CARE POINTS

- Common presenting complaint includes plantar heel pain first step out of bed in the morning or after periods of rest.
- Tissue bruising or edema near the origin or along the course of the plantar fascia may be indicative of a plantar fascial rupture or other injury.
- Gastrosoleal and plantar fascial specific stretching exercises with anti-inflammatory therapy (NSAIDs or injection) are the mainstay of treatment.

DISCLOSURE

Author has no pertinent disclosures for this subject matter.

REFERENCES

1. Snow SW, Bohne WH, DiCarlo E, et al. Anatomy of the Achilles tendon and plantar fascia in relation to the calcaneus in various age groups. Foot Ankle Int 1995;16:418–21.
2. Wearing SC, Smeathers JE, Urry SR, et al. The pathomechanics of plantar fasciitis. Sports Med 2006;36:585–611.
3. Sarafian SK. Anatomy of the foot and ankle: descriptive, topographic, functional. New York: JB Lippincott Company; 1983.
4. Beck CM, Dickerson AR, Kadado KJ, et al. Novel investigation of the deep band of the lateral plantar aponeurosis and its relationship with the lateral plantar nerve. Foot Ankle Int 2019;40(11):1325–30.
5. Hawkins Bj, Rangermen RJ Jr, Gibbons T, et al. An anatomic analysis of endoscopic plantar fascia release. Foot Ankle Int 1995;16:552–8.
6. Lin SC, Chen CPC, Tang SFT, et al. Stress distribution within the plantar aponeurosis during walking – a dynamic finite element analysis. J Mech Med Biol 2014;14(4):1450–3.
7. Benjamin M. The fascia of the limbs and back – a review. J Anat 2009;214:1018.

8. Stecco C, Corradin M, Macchi V, et al. Plantar fascia anatomy and its relationship with Achilles and paratenon. J Anat 2013;223:665–76.

9. Johal KS, Milner SA. Plantar fasciitis and the calcaneal spur: fact or fiction? Foot Ankle Surg 2012;18(1):39–41.

10. League AC. Current concepts review: plantar fasciitis. Foot Ankle Int 2008;29: 358–66.

11. Pohl MB, Hamill J, Davis IS. Biomechanical and anatomic factors associated with a history of plantar fasciitis in female runners. Clin J Sport Med 2009;19:372–6.

12. Riddle DL, Schappert SM. Volume of ambulatory care visits and patterns of care for patients diagnosed with plantar fasciitis: a national study of medical doctors. Foot Ankle Int 2004;25:303–10.

13. Sammarco GJ, Helfrey RB. Surgical treatment of recalcitrant plantar fasciitis. Foot Ankle Int 1996;17:520–6.

14. Thomas MJ, Roddy E, Zhang W, et al. The population prevalence of foot and ankle pain in middle and old age: a systematic review. Pain 2011;152:2870–80.

15. Lemont H, Ammirati KM, Usen N. Plantar fasciitis: a degenerative process (fasciosis) without inflammation. J Am Podiatr Med Assoc 2003;93:234–7.

16. Rompe JD, Hopf C, Nafe B, et al. Low-energy extracorporeal shock wave therapy for painful heel: a prospective controlled single-blind study. Arch Orthop Trauma Surg 1996;115:75–9.

17. Valizadeh MA, Afshar A, Hassani E, et al. Relationship between anthropometric findings and results of corticosteroid injections treatment in chronic plantar heel pain. Anesth Pain Med 2018;8:e64357.

18. Taunton JE, Ryban MB, Clement DB, et al. Plantar fasciitis: a retrospective analysis of 267 cases. Phys Ther Sport 2002;3:57–65.

19. Irving DB, Cook JL, Menz HB. Factors associated with chronic plantar heel pain: a systematic review. J Sci Med Sport 2006;9:11–24.

20. Pfeffer G, Bacchetti P, Deland J, et al. Comparison of custom and prefabricated orthoses in the initial treatment of proximal plantar fasciitis. Foot Ankle Int 1999; 20:214–21.

21. Porter MD, Shadbolt B. Intralesional corticosteroid injection versus extracorporeal shock wave therapy for plantar fasciopathy. Clin J Sport Med 2005;15:119–24.

22. Goff JD, Crawford R. Diagnosis and treatment of plantar fasciitis. Am Fam Physician 2011;84:676–82.

23. Tanz SS. Heel pain. Clin Orthop Relat Res 1963;28:169–78.

24. Forman WM, Green MA. The role of instrinsic musculature in the formation of inferior calcaneal exostoses. Clin Podiatr Med Surg 1990;7:217–23.

25. Zhou B, Zhou Y, Tao X, et al. Classification of calcaneal spurs and their relationship with plantar fasciitis. J Foot Ankle Surg 2015;454(4):594–600.

26. Schneider HP, Baca JM, Carpenter BB, et al. American college of foot and ankle surgeons clinical consensus statement: diagnosis and treatment of adult acquired infracalcaneal heel pain. J Foot Ankle Surg 2018;57:370–81.

27. Patel A, DiGiovanni B. Association between plantar fasciitis and isolated contracture of the gastrocnemius. Foot Ankle Int 2011;32(1):5–8.

28. Wenzel EM, Zajgana Z, Kelly KD, et al. Prevalence of equinus in patients diagnosed with plantar fasciitis. Foot Ankle Online J 2009;2(3):1.

29. DiGiovanni BF, Nawoczenski DA, Lintal ME, et al. Tissue-specific plantar fascia stretching exercise enhances outcomes in patients with chronic heel pain. A prospective, randomized study. JBJS 2003;856:1270–7.

30. DiGiovanni BF, Nawoczenski DA, Malay DP, et al. Plantar fascia-specific stretching exercise improves outcomes in patients with chronic plantar fasciitis. A prospective clinical trial with two-year follow-up. JBJS 2006;88(8):1775–81.
31. Barrett S, Erredge S. Growth factors for chronic plantar fasciitis? Podiatry Today 2004;17:37–42.
32. Peerbooms JC, Sluimer J, Bruijn D, et al. Positive effect of an autologous platelet concentrate in lateral epicondylitis in a double-blind randomized controlled trial: platelet-rich plasma versus corticosteroid injection with 1-year follow-up. Am J Sports Med 2010;38:255–62.
33. Ragab EMS, Othman AMA. Platelet rich plasma for treatment of chronic plantar fasciitis. Arch Orthop Trauma Surg 2012;132:1065–70.
34. Martinelli N, Marinozzi A, Carni S, et al. Platelet-rich plasma injections for chronic plantar fasciitis. Int Orthop 2013;37:839–42.
35. Mahintra P, Yamin M, Selhi HS, et al. Chronic plantar fasciitis: effect of platelet-rich plasma, corticosteroidm and placebo. Orthopedics 2016;39(32):e285–9.
36. Uygur E, Aktas B, Eceviz E, et al. Preliminary report on the role of dry needling verus corticosteroid injection, and effective treatment method for plantar fasciitis: a randomized controlled trial. J Foot Ankle Surf 2018;58:301–5.
37. Shetty SH, Dhond A, Arora M, et al. Platelet-rich plasma has better long-term results than corticosteroids or placebo for chronic plantar fasciitis: randomized control trial. J Foot Ankle Surg 2019;58:42–6.
38. Lee TG, Ahmad TS. Intralesional autologous blood injection compared to corticosteroid injection for treatment of chronic plantar fasciitis. A prospective, randomized controlled trial. Foot Ankle Intl 2007;28(9):984–90.
39. Tabrizi A, Dindarian S, Mohammadi S. The effect of corticosteroid local injection versus platelet-rich plasma for the treatment of plantar fasciitis in obese patients: a single-blind, randomized clinical trial. J Foot Ankle Surg 2020;59:64–8.
40. Alkhatib N, Salameh M, Ahmed AF, et al. Platelet-rich plasma versus corticosteroids in the treatment of chronic plantar fasciitis: a systematic review and meta-analysis of prospective comparative studies. Foot Ankle Surg 2020;59:546–52.
41. Ochiai N, Ohtori S, Sasho T, et al. Extracorporeal shock wave therapy improves motor dysfunction and pain originating from knee osteoarthritis in rats. Osteoarthritis Cartilage 2007;15:1093–6.
42. Berta L, Fazzari A, Ficco AM, et al. Extracorporeal shock waves enhance normal fibroblast proliferation in vitro and activate mRNA expression for TGF-beta1 and for collagen types I and III. Acta Orthop 2009;80:612–7.
43. Rompe JD, Schoellner C, Nafe B. Evaluation of low-energy extracorporeal shock-wave application for treatment of chronic plantar fasciitis. JBJS 2002;84(3):335–41.
44. Ugurlar M, Sonmez MM, Ugurlar OY, et al. Effectiveness of four different treatment modalities in the treatment of chronic plantar fasciitis during a 36-month follow-up period: a randomized controlled trial. J Foot Ankle Surg 2018;57:913–8.
45. Mardani-Kivi M, Mobarakeh MK, Hassanzadeh Z, et al. Treatment outcomes of corticosteroid injection and extracorporeal shcok wave therapy as two primary therapeutic methods for acute plantar fasciitis: a prospective randomized clinic trial. Foot Ankle Surg 2015;54:1047–52.
46. Moneagudo M, Maceira E, Garcia-Virto V, et al. Chronic plantar fasciitis: plantar fasciotomy versus gastrocnemius recession. Intl Orthop 2013;37:1845–50.
47. Barrett S, Day S. Endoscopic plantar fasciotomy for chronic plantar fasciitis/heel spur syndrome: surgical technique – early clinical results. J Foot Surg 1990;30:568–70.

48. Barrett SL, Day SV, Pignetti T, et al. Endoscopic plantar fasciotomy: a multi-surgeon prospective analysis of 652 cases. J Foot Ankle Surg 1995;34:400–6.
49. Tomczak RL, Haverstock BD. A retrospective comparison of endoscopic plantar fasciotomy to open plantar fasciotomy with heel spur resection for chronic plantar fasciitis/heel spur syndrome. J Foot Ankle Surg 1995;34(3):305–11.
50. O'Malley MJ, Page A, Cook R. Endoscopic plantar fasciotomy for chronic heel pain. Foot Ankle Int 2000;21(6):505–10.
51. Cottom JM, Maker JM. Endoscopic debridement for treatment of chronic plantar fasciitis: an innovative surgical technique. J Foot Ankle Surg 2016;55:655–8.
52. Tangh Y, Deng P, Wang G, et al. The clinical efficacy of two endoscopic surgical approaches for intractable plantar fasciitis. J Foot Ankle Surg 2020;59:280–5.
53. Singh D, Angel JH, Bentley G, et al. Fortnightly review. Plantar fasciitis. BMJ 1997;315(7101):172–5.
54. Young CC, Rutherford DS, Niedfeldt MW. Treatment of plantar fasciitis. Am Fam Physician 2001;63:467–78.
55. Martin RL, Irrgang JJ, Conti SF. Outcome study of subjects with insertional plantar fasciitis. Foot Ankle Int 1998;19:803–11.
56. Gill LH, Liebzak GM. Outcome of nonsurgical treatment for plantar fasciitis. Foot Ankle Int 1996;17:527–32.
57. Wolgin M, Cook C, Graham C, et al. Conservative treatment of plantar heel pain: long term follow-up. Foot Ankle Int 1994;15:97–102.

Acute Achilles Tendon Ruptures

Donald Buddecke Jr, DPM

KEYWORDS

- Achilles • Achilles tendon • Achilles tendon rupture

KEY POINTS

- There is an evolution, with more surgeons utilizing an aggressive functional rehabilitation with conservative management.
- Surgical intervention still is the treatment of choice for elite-level athletes.
- The treatment of choice for patient populations other than elite athletes is an ever-evolving decision and remains an individual choice between patient and physician.

The Achilles tendon is the hardest working tendon in the human body. This largest and strongest tendon also is the tendon most frequently injured.[1] Considering the number of steps that are taken throughout the day and the added stress through the tendon during exercise, this structure is asked to sustain a tremendous amount of force with these activities. Consequently, it is not surprising that injuries to this tendon are common.

There is an ever-evolving debate about the best treatment option for Achilles tendon ruptures. There was a relative consensus that operative treatment yielded the best outcomes. Much of this is based on results in athletic populations. Conservative treatment was considered only for the elderly and those with very inactive lifestyles. There has been an evolution, however, with more surgeons utilizing an aggressive functional rehabilitation with conservative management. Surgical intervention still is the treatment of choice for elite-level athletes. The treatment of choice for patient populations other than elite athletes is an ever-evolving decision and remains an individual choice between patient and physician.

INCIDENCE AND DEMOGRAPHICS

As the population continues to age, yet continues to remain highly active, ruptures of the Achilles tendon are on the rise. The incidence of Achilles ruptures in the United States has increased from 0.67/10,000 people in 2005 to 1.08/10,000 people in 2011.[2] These authors did attribute this significant increase to an aging population

Private Practice, Foot and Ankle Surgery, Foot & Ankle Specialists, 18010 R Plaza, Omaha, NE 68135, USA
E-mail address: debuddecke@yahoo.com

Clin Podiatr Med Surg 38 (2021) 201–226
https://doi.org/10.1016/j.cpm.2020.12.006
0891-8422/21/© 2021 Elsevier Inc. All rights reserved.

podiatric.theclinics.com

that continues to be physically active. A retrospective review of a 20-year period in Denmark also demonstrated a significant increase in incidence of Achilles ruptures.[3] This is a particularly good reflection of the true incidence due to the free health care in Denmark along with the requirements for all to be registered in the country. These authors saw an increase of Achilles ruptures from 26.95/100,000 in 1994 to 31.17/100,000 in 2013. There was a significant increase in those greater than 50 years of age whereas those from 30 years to 50 years of age saw no increase and those 18 years to 30 years of age saw a decrease. There also has been seasonal variation of the injury. This tends to occur when the population starts to become active. This has been shown to occur in the spring with peak incidence occurring in March.[4,5] An increased incidence, however, was noted in the fall, with a peak in the month of September in the Denmark study. All major sports are started after summer in this country, likely accounting for this variation.

This injury is seen overwhelmingly in the fifth decade of life. Raikin and colleagues[6] showed an average age of 46.4 in men and a slightly older age in women (50.0 years of age). Ganestam and colleagues[3] demonstrated a mean age in men and women of 42 years of age in 1994, which increased to 49 years of age (men) and 48 (women) in 2013. Middle-aged men make up the largest demographic that sustain an Achilles rupture.[6,7] The male-to-female ratio is significant. One study demonstrated a 5.39:1 ratio of men to women in acute ruptures.[8] Other studies have shown a ratio from 1.67:1 to 6.90:1.[3–5,9–15] Is this a result of men having more relative muscle mass than women, or are there hormonal differences causing this discrepancy? It has been shown that women had a higher rate of general musculoskeletal injuries than men.[16] Yet, Achilles tendon rupture is male dominated. It appears that ligament injuries are more common than musculotendinous injuries in female athletes. Wojtys and colleagues[17] demonstrated an increased incidence of ACL ruptures in women during the ovulatory phase of menstrual cycle when estrogen levels were higher. Later it was noted that oral contraceptives appeared to blunt the injury spike seen with ovulation.[18] So, why is the rate of Achilles ruptures significantly less than in men? Other studies have shown no difference in the mechanical properties within the tendon with fluctuations in female sex hormones.[19–21] Still another study suggested that chronic exposure of estrogen leads to less Achilles strain.[22] Additionally, it has been demonstrated that female sex hormones have an inhibitory effect on muscle fiber diameter.[23] Consequently, this could support the theory that the relative increase in muscle mass and increased fiber diameter in men make this a much more common occurrence in the male population.

More athletic events being televised along with high-definition broadcasting has allowed witnessing various sporting injuries, including slow motion analysis of Achilles tendon ruptures. Numerous elite-level athletes have video demonstrating the moment of their Achilles rupture. This shows the moment that eccentric contracture takes place and the eventual loss of integrity of the tendon unit as it ruptures. The power that is placed through this contracting muscle unit as the tendon stretches eventually leads to failure in the diseased tendon. In a normal and healthy tendon, the rupture at the tendon probably does not occur. Instead, if failure is going to take place in the presence of a healthy tendon, it generally occurs at the musculotendinous junction. In the older population, failure tends to occur at the tendon insertion site on bone. The location of the rupture occurs at the area of tendon disease, which does correspond to the watershed area of the tendon (2–8 cm proximal to the insertion site). Excessive use with microtrauma occurring in this location places the tendon at risk. The persistent microtrauma with limited healing ability because of the watershed area and the increased activity level makes this a troubling cycle.

Although usually the result of athletic injury, Achilles ruptures can occur even with normal everyday activities (ie, stepping off a curb or going up a flight of stairs). Various studies have demonstrated a high rate of acute ruptures caused by athletic events. Rates of Achilles ruptures caused by athletic activity have ranged from 59% to 81%.[3–6,9–13] As discussed previously, it generally is accepted that healthy tendons are not at risk for rupture. It is likely that damage has been done with repetitive use and microtrauma, and an inciting event leads to the eventual rupture. Histologic degeneration has been reported at Achilles tendon rupture sites.[24] Additionally, a study revealed a high incidence (865 cases over a 3-year period) of Achilles ruptures in the United States military, suggesting likely overuse problems that eventually lead to rupture.[25]

DIAGNOSIS

The Achilles tendon easily is examined due to its superficial nature. Injuries to the area are not hard to diagnose and ruptures are suspected easily. Typically, there is significant edema compared with the contralateral ankle (**Fig. 1**). Patients describe a pain at the back of the ankle and often state they felt like they got kicked or that something hit them in the back of the ankle. It is not overly painful, but it is the surprise of the situation that stuns them. These patients generally present to an urgent care facility or emergency department and often they are immobilized and referred for definitive care. They can be referred with an accurate diagnosis of Achilles rupture or just as an ankle injury if partial rupture is present. Consequently, they often are delayed in presentation to a specialist's office for 1 week or 2 weeks.

Clinically, the muscle groups can be assessed, usually with only a little discomfort to the patient. Weakness can be noted but there can be some plantarflexion strength because the plantarflexors are able to function fully. The Thompson test can be reliable with complete ruptures. If full rupture is present, the foot does not plantarflex while squeezing the calf muscle (**Fig. 2**). There typically is a dramatic difference from the contralateral limb. The amount of tension on the foot also can be assessed and is diminished considerably on the injured limb (**Fig. 3**). With the patient lying prone, flex the knees to 90° and compare the injured limb with the uninjured. With complete ruptures, the foot usually is parallel to the ground while the uninjured limb shows some

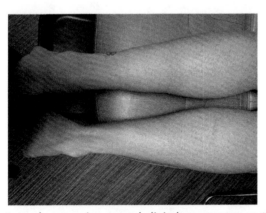

Fig. 1. Clinical photograph comparing normal clinical appearance on the right with the typical appearance after an Achilles rupture on the right. Notice the lack of Achilles definition on the left ankle and the lack of plantarflexion tone compared with the uninjured right ankle.

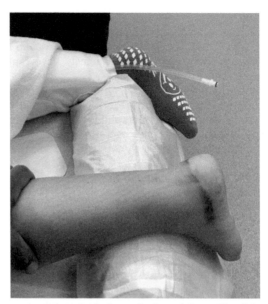

Fig. 2. Positive Thompson test: lack of plantarflexion of the ankle while squeezing the calf.

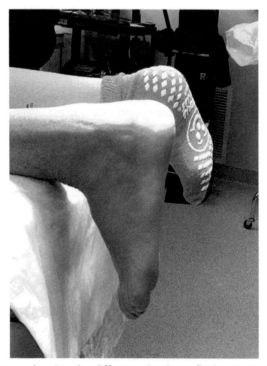

Fig. 3. Clinical pictures showing the difference in plantarflexion tone of an injured ankle compared to the contralateral normal ankle. Notice the resting plantarflexion tone of the uninjured side and the lack of plantarflexion of the injured extremity.

plantarflexion (**Figs. 4** and **5**). There even can be some discrepancy in plantarflexion tone with just having the patient lying prone or supine (**Fig. 6**). Because this tendon sits subcutaneously, a palpable defect often can be detected (**Figs. 7** and **8**). A combination of a positive Thompson test, asymmetry with resting tension of the ankles, and palpable defect makes a clinical diagnosis relatively easy to make.

If these clinical scenarios are not definitive, additional diagnostic modalities can be implemented. Ultrasound is a viable option. Again, due to its superficial nature, the Achilles tendon is amenable to ultrasound examination. Ruptures and some partial ruptures can be diagnosed easily. Ultrasound does not offer a good overall picture, however, of the integrity of the surrounding tendon. Magnetic resonance imaging (MRI) is a valuable tool when complete rupture is not obvious. This gives the advantage of a complete diagnosis of partial or complete rupture in addition to providing valuable information regarding the health of the tendon proximally and distally. This can aid in determining the best treatment option and the best recovery protocol. Although MRI evaluation is not mandatory for all these injuries, is remains a valuable tool without any harm to the patient (**Figs. 9–12**).

TREATMENT

Conservative treatment of Achilles tendon ruptures was relatively common a few decades ago. Less than satisfactory outcomes were experienced, however, due to weakness and reruptures. As a result, there was a transition to surgical intervention. This generally included extensive incisions for open repair. Although the strength was better and reruptures rates diminished, there were various complications that pushed for other less invasive techniques. Wound healing issues, infection, and adhesions were some of the main complications encountered with extensive open

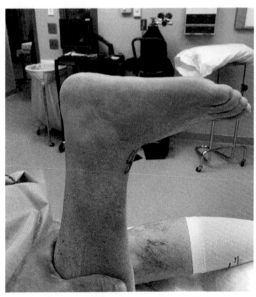

Fig. 4. Clinical pictures showing the difference in plantarflexion tone of an injured ankle compared to the contralateral normal ankle. Notice the resting plantarflexion tone of the uninjured side and the lack of plantarflexion of the injured extremity.

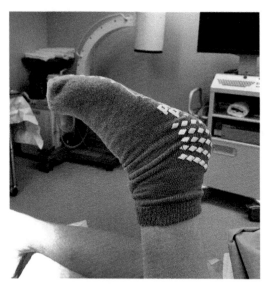

Fig. 5. Clinical pictures showing the difference in plantarflexion tone of an injured ankle compared to the contralateral normal ankle. Notice the resting plantarflexion tone of the uninjured side and the lack of plantarflexion of the injured extremity.

procedures. Percutaneous techniques and minimally invasive techniques have evolved in an attempt to preserve strength, minimize reruptures, and prevent open wounds and adhesions.

Nonoperative Treatment

The advantages of nonoperative treatment include minimal concerns for infection or adhesions, not to mention that patients do not have to go through a surgical process.

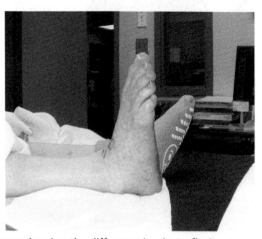

Fig. 6. Clinical pictures showing the difference in plantarflexion tone of an injured ankle compared to the contralateral normal ankle. Notice the resting plantarflexion tone of the uninjured side and the lack of plantarflexion of the injured extremity.

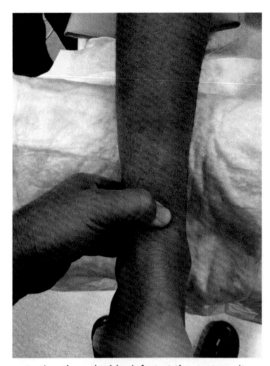

Fig. 7. Picture demonstrating the palpable defect at the rupture site.

The disadvantages generally include a higher rerupture rate, need for adherence to a strict rehabilitation protocol, weakness, and prolonged healing times. It has been demonstrated that surgical intervention can provide a superior outcome compared with conservative treatment. The details of conservative treatment, however, are important. Nonoperative treatment that includes long-term cast immobilization generally do not have a better outcome than surgery. The best nonsurgical treatment includes various forms of functional rehabilitation, including early range of motion and early weight-bearing activities. With an extremely strict rehabilitation protocol, several studies have demonstrated decreased rerupture rates with conservative treatment.[14,26–32] Zhou and colleagues[33] demonstrated similar rerupture rates with surgical and conservative treatment if early functional rehabilitation is implemented. The details of functional rehabilitation can vary from early range of motion to early weight bearing. Typically, there is a cast or splint applied with ankle in plantarflexion (approximately 30°) for 7 days to 10 days. At that point, patient is placed into a removable walking boot and allowed early range of motion or weight bearing in a controlled ankle motion (CAM) boot with heel wedges. Once weight bearing is implemented, the wedges are removed every 4 days to 8 days until ankle is in neutral. Weight bearing continues and often functional rehabilitation with physical therapy is instituted. Often, the patient is out of the CAM boot at 6 weeks to 8 weeks.

There certainly are limitations when conservative management is desired. As described previously, presentation of these injuries often is delayed. If the diagnosis is delayed too long (7–14 days), conservative treatment no longer may be an option. The importance of conservative management is being able to plantarflex the foot and allow the ruptured ends to come together. Patients with Achilles ruptures often

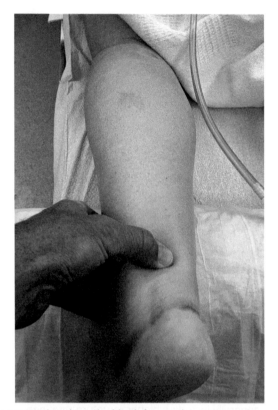

Fig. 8. Picture demonstrating the palpable defect at the rupture site.

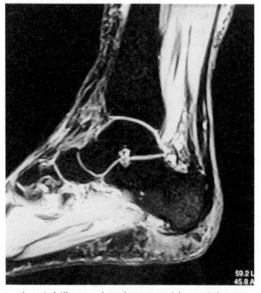

Fig. 9. MRI demonstrating Achilles tendon damage with partial rupture.

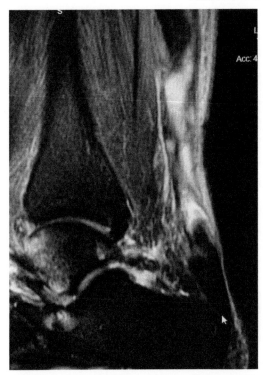

Fig. 10. MRI demonstrating complete Achilles tendon rupture with significant gap at the rupture site.

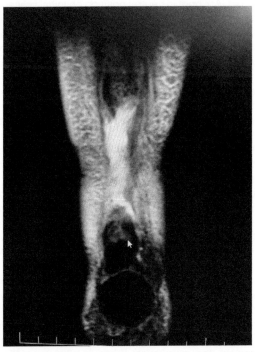

Fig. 11. MRI demonstrating complete Achilles tendon rupture with significant gap at the rupture site.

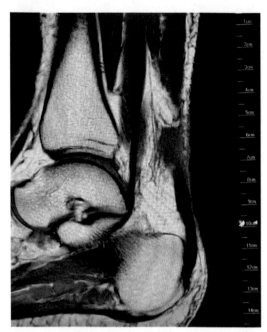

Fig. 12. MRI demonstrating complete Achilles tendon rupture with significant gap at the rupture site.

are placed in a splint or CAM boot in neutral position on initial presentation in an urgent care facility or emergency department. If a patient was not placed in significant plantarflexion, the gap between the tendon ends persists. With a delay of 1 week to 2 weeks, scar tissue and fibrous tissue already has filled the gap and appropriate apposition is not possible. Cetti and colleagues[34] described the average separation of the rupture site as 2.7 cm. This can be exacerbated by neutral positioning of the limb in a splint or cast. Not all Achilles ruptures are able to be approximated with plantarflexion alone. Although there are promising studies for conservative treatment, the limiting factor is the ability to get the ruptured ends in close apposition at the start of treatment.

In those cases of immediate diagnosis made and it is decided to implement conservative treatment, strict rehabilitation is the next obstacle to attain a good outcome. Patient compliance is paramount. As with every aspect of medicine, education of the patient is critical. Understanding the steps utilized and the rationale can be helpful in maintaining compliance throughout the course of treatment. When that happens, success can be achieved. In a randomized controlled trial, conservative treatment was compared with percutaneous and open repair.[35] Conservative treatment consisted of immediate casting at 30° of plantarflexion for 10 days. CAM boot then was applied in gravity equinus and weight bearing was allowed after 8 days. Wedges were removed every 4 days. Strengthening rehabilitation was implemented at 6 weeks. Calf circumference was slightly lower in the conservative group. When comparing the 2 sides, equal strength was noted in conservative group whereas 1 patient in each of the surgical groups showed a decrease in strength. One patient in each group did not return to sport. No reruptures were noted in any of the groups. Patients reported 91% excellent satisfaction in the conservative group, 72% excellent satisfaction in percutaneous group, and 83% excellent satisfaction in the open group. Only 9/34 patients in this study group performed sport at a high intensity prior to surgery and there were no elite athletes in this study population. A study from China completed a meta-analysis of randomized controlled trials comparing surgical with nonsurgical treatment of Achilles ruptures.[34] This included 10 randomized controlled trials with approximately 1000 patients. Rerupture was noted in 11.04% of nonsurgical patients and 4.24% of surgical patients. When eliminating reruptures, however, the complication rates of surgical versus nonsurgical patients were 28.47% and 6.91%, respectively. There was a slight advantage of functional outcomes in the surgical group but no significance with regard to return to sport. This study found that there was a lower rerupture rate in the nonsurgical group if early functional rehabilitation was implemented whereas the opposite was noted if early functional rehabilitation was not implemented. Similarly, Soroceanu and colleagues[36] found a lower rerupture rate in nonoperative treatment of Achilles ruptures if early functional rehabilitation was implemented.

Operative Treatment

Surgical treatment of Achilles tendon ruptures generally can be broken down into open repair, percutaneous repair, and minimally invasive repair. In many of the reported studies, percutaneous repair and minimally invasive repair often are used interchangeably and not separated when data are reported. It appears that minimally invasive repair is more prevalent to true percutaneous repair. The repair construct and some of the modifications have allowed this to be much stronger than true percutaneous repair techniques.

OPEN REPAIR

Although open repair still is used, there is a trend at less invasive options. Open repair offers the advantage of complete visualization of proximal and distal stumps of the tendon. This allows the ability to gain a strong suture construct and directly visualize the apposition of tendon ends. The ankle then can be taken through range of motion while observing the strength of repair. This offers the additional advantage of less creep that can be common in minimally invasive techniques. This postrepair lengthening has been attributed to suture creep and suture failure that can be concerns with poor tendon quality proximal and distal to rupture site. With open procedures, it typically is easier to grab more tendon and healthier tendon to prevent this problem.

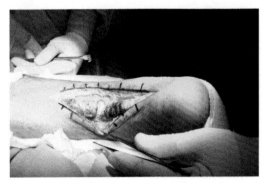

Fig. 13. Intraoperative photograph showing open Achilles tendon repair with Krackow suture technique.

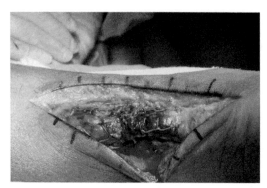

Fig. 14. Intraoperative photograph showing open Achilles tendon repair with Krackow suture technique.

The ability for surgeons to choose the suturing technique they desire is another advantage. Limits are placed with percutaneous and minimally invasive techniques (**Figs. 13–15**).

The drawback to open repair always has been the concern for dehiscence and adhesions. This tendon is superficial, and no padding is available once the skin is closed. Even with meticulous technique, the paratenon has some damage and can be difficult to get adequate repair. If wound dehiscence occurs, the tendon repair site is exposed

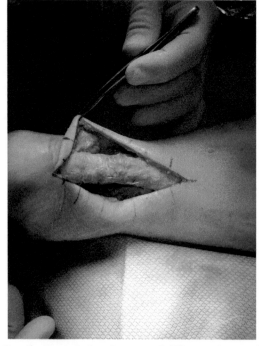

Fig. 15. Intraoperative photograph showing open Achilles tendon repair with Krackow suture technique.

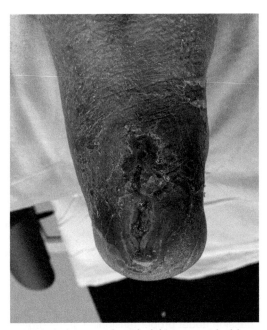

Fig. 16. Postoperative clinical photograph with dehiscence at incision area.

and at risk for devitalization and infection. If the wound does heal, many times there are adhesions encountered that can be debilitating to the patient. This also can lead to less than desirable cosmesis (**Fig. 16**).

More dissection that leads to more tissue disruption also increases the risk of infection. As wound healing becomes difficult, dehiscence is encountered. The longer the wound is open in a relatively devitalized area, the risk of infection rises. Additionally, the foreign material used for the repair decreases the amount of bacterial load needed to cause an infection. Consequently, there is motivation to find less-invasive options.

Specific suturing techniques have been described and studied. Additionally, the type and size of suture material are debated. These various suturing techniques have been a focus of study to determine the strongest construct. Watson and colleagues[37] compared the Krackow, Kessler, and Bunnell techniques. These investigators concluded that the Krackow stitch was superior. A later study comparing the triple-bundle technique to the Krackow method demonstrated an increase in strength of the triple-bundle technique.[38] These investigators felt that the increased number of strands across the repair site and the fact that suture knots were away from the repair site were beneficial. Additionally, a cadaveric study compared sutures tied at repair site (Krackow stitch) with sutures tied away from the repair site (gift box modification of the Krackow technique).[39] Force to failure was significantly larger in the gift box modification. Other investigators have shown no difference in strength when comparing double-Bunnell, double-Kessler, and double-Krackow.[40] The apprehension with some of these suturing techniques as surgeons try to increase strength is the concern of tendon strangulation.

The other component of these repair techniques is the type and size of suture material. Backus and colleagues[41] evaluated various repairs with FiberWire (Arthrex, Naples, Florida) and FiberTape (Arthrex) compared with 2-0 suture. The control was 6 strands of No. 2 FiberWire. This was compared with 1 technique using 4 of 6 strands using no. 2 FiberWire and 2 of 6 strands using 2-mm FiberTape (2T technique), another technique using no. 2 FiberWire for 2 of 6 strands and 2-mm FiberTape for 4 of 6 strands (4T technique), and the final technique using 2-0 suture with double 6-strand (12 core strands [12S] technique). The conclusion was that the 2T and 12S techniques showed the best survival with cycles to failure and load to failure. Most of the failures occurred at the knot and this was even more concerning with FiberTape. Additionally, with the addition of more FiberTape strands, there was concern for a sawing through the tendon as mode of failure. Yet another study comparing FiberWire to FiberTape was performed.[42] These investigators compared Mason-Allen, whipstitch, and Krackow stitches using these 2 suture options. They noted pull-through as the most common mode of failure with a slight advantage to FiberWire over FiberTape.

Various considerations need to be weighed when determining the best type and size of suture. Generally speaking, a no. 2 or 2-0 stitch is common for the Achilles tendon. Suture size and type certainly is a major consideration for the Achilles because the number of core strands and the suture caliber has been shown to significantly affect the strength of flexor repair in the forearm.[43] A nonabsorbable stitch usually is used to maintain strength throughout the rehabilitation process. The concern if not using a braided stitch is the increase potential for suture creep whereas braided suture can grasp the tendon more effectively as healing takes place. These same concepts hold true for percutaneous treatment and minimally invasive treatment. The size of the sutures is somewhat limited with the use of jigs.

There is some discussion about proper tensioning of the repair. Many reports talk about evaluating the resting position of the contralateral limb and applying tension to the repair to match that limb. The gap in tendon ends and the contracture of the calf muscle, however, are different in every case. So, the goal should be to approximate the tendon ends. Typically, this leads to significant plantarflexion of the ankle after the repair. This plantarflexion is the goal after Achilles repair (**Fig. 17**). This ensures good tension of the repair and hopefully prevents elongation. Future rehabilitation allows a return of flexibility of the triceps surae once healing is complete. In contrast, if a repair is in a lengthened position, recovery is difficult, and weakness is the result.

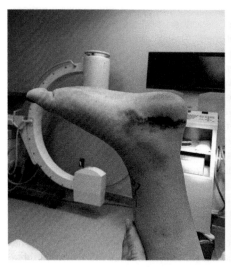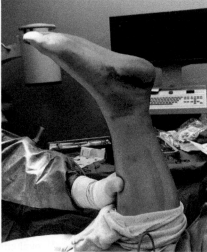

Fig. 17. Intraoperative pictures comparing the plantarflexion of the ankle before and after Achilles repair. The repair is placed at maximum plantarflexion.

PERCUTANEOUS REPAIR

True percutaneous techniques have been described. Ma and Griffith[44] described their technique in 1977. This includes stab incisions on the medial and lateral aspects of the tendon. Needles with suture attached are placed through these stab holes and placed through the tendon in varying transverse and diagonal paths. This is done proximally and distally, and the tendon ends are brought together. The obvious advantage is the limited disruption of the soft tissue around the rupture site. Theoretically, this keeps the hematoma, along with the healing biology, intact to allow a quicker recovery. Wound dehiscence and infection are minimized. The disadvantage of percutaneous repair is the inability to visualize the repair directly. Limited exposure also makes the repair potentially weaker because limited suturing techniques are available with percutaneous repair and concerns for appropriate tendon capture.

MINIMALLY INVASIVE REPAIR

An attempt to get the best of both open and percutaneous repair lead to the development of minimally invasive techniques. Jigs, such as the Achillon (Integra, Plainsboro, New Jersey) and PARS device (Arthrex), have been developed to aid with this process. The goal was to incorporate the advantages of open and percutaneous procedures and minimize the disadvantages of each of the techniques. With minimally invasive techniques, a small incision is made at the rupture site. This allows direct visualization of the repair and augmentation of the repair, if deemed necessary. The potential downside is removal of the hematoma and the biology from the area of repair. The limited dissection proximal and distal to the rupture leads to less scarring and adhesions and less concern for dehiscence and infection. The jig concept allows better and stronger suturing techniques. Tendon capture is still a concern, however, when compared with open techniques. Tendon capture concerns is more notable in patients with larger body mass index (BMI).[45] Rerupture rates after minimally invasive techniques have been reported, from 0% to 16.7%[46–54] (**Figs. 18–25**).

COMPARISONS

Several randomized controlled trials have shown that surgical treatment of Achilles ruptures can reduce the rerupture risk compared with conservative treatment. Surgical treatment, however, tends to lead to higher complication rates.[26,33,46,55–59] As discussed previously, the incidence of Achilles ruptures is increasing. There is a trend, however, toward a decrease in surgical intervention as functional rehabilitation becomes more popular.[60] Still, surgical intervention typically is favored in the athletic population. This certainly is the case in the elite athlete but also a favored option in those patients with a desire to remain highly active. It has been shown that surgical intervention allows a faster return to work compared with nonsurgical treatment.[26,37,61] Additionally, a level 1 study by Lantto and colleagues[62] suggested that operative repair increases strength and improves clinical outcomes at 6 months and 18 months. There are other studies showing evidence that surgical repair reduces strength discrepancies[63] and improves plantarflexion function.[27]

A recent study with computer generated randomization compared open technique (double-Bunnell stitch) to percutaneous (Ma and Griffith technique) and nonsurgical treatment.[64] Rehabilitation was the same for all groups, including non–weight-bearing cast for 10 days, then placed in equinus in CAM boot and allowed weight bearing. Wedges were removed every 4 days. Active rehabilitation was implemented at 6 weeks and CAM boot was discontinued. These investigators conclude that nonsurgical

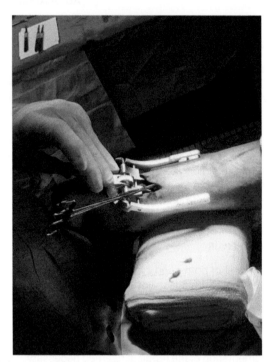

Fig. 18. Minimally invasive technique with PARS device in place and clamp placed on proximal stump.

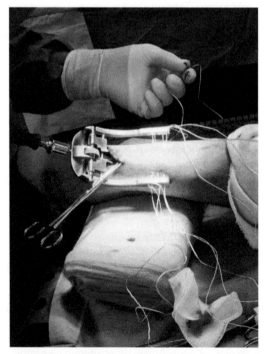

Fig. 19. Sutures have been placed through the jig and into the proximal stump of the Achilles tendon.

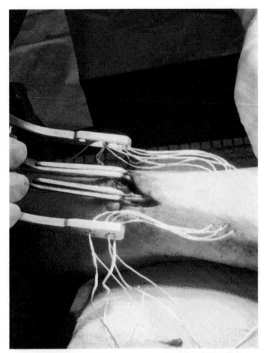

Fig. 20. The jig is retracted gently, and the sutures are brought into the wound.

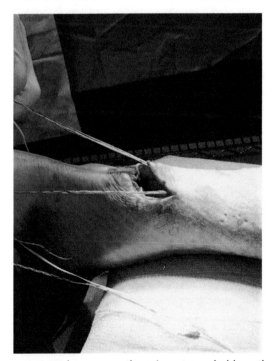

Fig. 21. The sutures are tested to ensure there is a strong hold on the Achilles tendon. Often, these individual stands are loaded after locking the sutures. This includes gentle traction while sliding back and forth through the tendon. This helps prevent future creep of the suture.

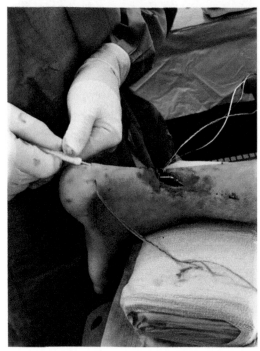

Fig. 22. A suture passer is placed from the insertion site area through the distal stump and into the rupture site. The sutures then are passed into the distal stump and out the stab incision.

treatment was just as effective as surgical treatment in a majority of patients. Deng and colleagues[65] noted no significant difference with return to sport with a meta-analysis of randomized controlled trials comparing surgical with nonsurgical treatment. Nonsurgical patients, however, have rerupture rates of 9.8% compared with 3.7%

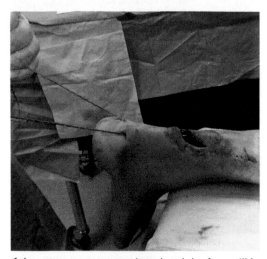

Fig. 23. Both sides of the suture are now tensioned and the foot will be plantarflexed. This maneuver will bring the rupture site together.

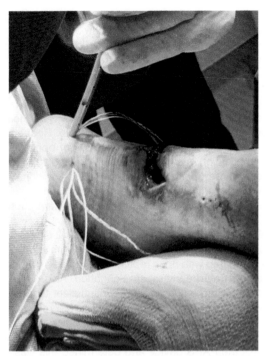

Fig. 24. The sutures then are anchored into the calcaneus while the foot is plantarflexed. The rupture site can then be augmented with additional suture if desired.

in the surgical group. Yet another meta-analysis studied surgical and nonsurgical treatment.[33] These investigators also showed a higher rerupture rate with nonsurgical treatment (11.4% vs 4.24%, respectively). They noted, however, that studies that implemented early weight bearing (within 2 weeks) for nonsurgical care versus just

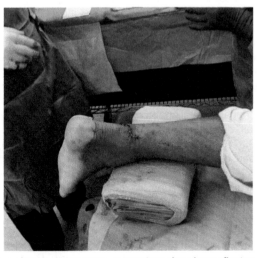

Fig. 25. After incision closure, it is easy to appreciate the plantarflexion of the foot, return of tension to the Achilles, and the wrinkles on the back of the ankle.

early range of motion showed fewer reruptures than the surgical group. The overall complication rate with surgery was 28.47% compared with only 6.91% in the nonsurgical group. Surgical patients did do better with functional outcome, as noted with better results in 2 jump tests and 1 muscular endurance test.

Comparing the PARS technique to open technique has been popular.[54,66] One study compared 169 open procedures (Krackow stitch) to 101 PARS cases. Return to baseline activity at 5 months was noted in 98% of PARS cases versus 82% of open cases. No reruptures were noted in either group. Sural neuritis was noted in 3.0% of open procedures and none of the PARS group. Reoperation was noted in 2% of PARS cases for FiberWire reaction and 1.8% of open procedures for deep infection. Overall complication rate was 5.0% for PARS and 10.6% for open.[54] Cottom and colleagues[66] compared open (Krackow) to PARS. Additionally, these investigators compared PARS proximally with suture anchor attachment into the calcaneus distally (knotless technique). This knotless technique did turn out to be the strongest construct.

A biomechanical comparison evaluating open repair to 2 different minimally invasive techniques was performed. Achillon, PARS, and PARS with suture anchor attachment to calcaneus were compared with open repair.[45] The concern was that minimally invasive techniques demonstrated early repair elongation. Also, there was concern that these techniques made it more susceptible to insufficient tendon capture. This was most concerning with larger BMIs. Ultimate strength to failure, however, was equal between the open and minimally invasive groups. Another study compared the 2 jig options (Achillon and PARS) for minimally invasive Achilles repair.[67] These investigators showed superiority of the PARS device and determined this was due to the locking ability of the sutures with the PARS device. Without the locking ability of the sutures, the Achillon device had the tendency to pull through the tendon. The PARS failure was due to suture failure.

COMPLICATIONS

The surgical, such as rerupture, adhesions, dehiscence, infection, and sural nerve injury, have been discussed. It has been reported that open repair can be associated with 27% complications rate.[59] Another study looking at overall complication rate demonstrated 30.4% with open procedures, 15.3% with nonsurgical treatment, and 10.3% with minimally invasive techniques.[46] Still another study showed a complication rate of 9.7% with minimally invasive techniques compared with 21% with open treatment.[53] A more recent report reported on complications with open and minimally invasive techniques.[68] They noted wound infection in 2.8%, sural nerve issue in 0.42%, dehiscence in 0.09%, and deep vein thrombosis (DVT) in 0.97% of surgical and 1.2% of nonsurgical cases. Another study that looked at complications of minimally invasive repair did show 5.18% of sural nerve issues. Superficial infection (0.37%) and DVT (0.37%) rates, however, were extremely low.[69] Higher complication rates also have been described. Complications after minimally invasive treatment have been documented, with 19% sural nerve issues and even 8% rerupture.[61] Other studies have shown sural nerve injury, ranging from 9% to 18%.[70,71] Many of the reports, however, demonstrate a successful resolution of sural nerve problems over time. One of the biggest concerns with minimally invasive procedures was the sural nerve injury possibilities and less satisfactory outcomes. Sural nerve injuries do not appear to be a major concern. It has been demonstrated that this minimally invasive approach can have a significantly reduced risk of superficial wound infection and produce 3-times greater patient satisfaction compared with open procedures.[72] Still others have demonstrated better functional outcomes while showing fewer complications with minimally invasive treatment.[73,74] The recent trend is that minimally invasive techniques are not burdened with extensive sural nerve issues. If they are encountered, they tend to resolve with time.

Meta-analysis studies have demonstrated a deep infection rate of 2.36% with open repair.[59,75] The overall infection rate for percutaneous repair has ranged from 0% to 13.3%.[44,46,47,52–54,76,77] Foreign body reaction has been described.[54,78,79] Some of these suture materials are designed to provide significant strength for repair and minimize creep through the tendon. As a result, an increased inflammatory response or even foreign body reaction can occur.

Venous thromboembolism continues to be a major concern with foot and ankle injuries. The limited mobility that can occur after an Achilles rupture should add concern to those treating this problem. There have been high DVT rates reported, including a 34% rate of DVT and 3% rate of pulmonary embolism in 95 cases.[27] Healy and colleagues[80] reported a 6.3% incidence of symptomatic thrombosis and Calder and colleagues[81] reported an incidence of 7%. Venous thromboembolism is not documented as a high-volume complication in Achilles ruptures, whether treated conservatively or surgically. The overall incidence rates of venous thromboembolism in foot and ankle surgery are 0.6% and 1% with and without chemoprophylaxis, respectively.[82] It is a complication, however, that can have dire consequences if it leads to pulmonary embolus. It should be discussed with every patient and appropriate prophylaxis implemented if risk factors are significant.

CHRONIC ACHILLES RUPTURE

Neglected Achilles tendons or those that are unsuccessfully treated conservatively can cause chronic problems. Weakness with limited function can result. Surgical intervention for this problem is often addresses differently than the acute injury. This chronic problem generally requires a flexor hallucis longus (FHL) transfer or gastrocnemius lengthening and turn down flap. The FHL transfer is utilized to add some vascularity from the FHL muscle belly to the relatively minimally vascular repair site. Additionally, this transfer can provide some additional strength and function. The gastrocnemius recession allows the ruptured ends a chance to be brought together and the turn down can add strength to the repair site. Consequently, these approaches for chronic ruptures amenable to minimally invasive approaches. This chronic problem is mentioned for completeness but is a separate topic and is not the basis of this article.

CLINICS CARE POINTS

- Acute Achilles ruptures should be treated based on the specifics of the individual patient.
- Surgical and non-surgical treatment may be appropriate if specific details are followed.

REFERENCES

1. Calleja M, Connell DA. The achilles tendon. Semin Musculoskelet Radiol 2010;14: 307–22.
2. Erickson BJ, Cvetanovich GL, Nwachukwu BU, et al. Trends in the management of Achilles tendon ruptures in the United States Medicare population, 2005-2011. Orthop J Sports Med 2014;2:1–6.

3. Ganestam A, Kallemose T, Troelsen A, et al. Increasing incidence of acute Achilles tendon rupture and a noticeable decline in surgical treatment from 1994 to 2013: a nationwide registry study of 33,160 patients. Knee Surg Sports Traumatol Arthrosc 2016;24:3730–7.

4. Nyyssonen T, Luthje P, Kroger H. The increasing incidence and difference in sex distribution of Achilles tendon rupture in Finland in 1987-1999. Scand J Surg 2008;97:272–5.

5. Suchak AA, Bostick G, Reid D, et al. The incidence of Achilles tendon ruptures in Edmonton, Canada. Foot Ankle Int 2005;26:932–6.

6. Raikin SM, Garras DN, Krapchev PV. Achilles tendon injuries in a United States population. Foot Ankle Int 2013;34:475–80.

7. Soldatis JJ, Goodfellow DB, Wilber JH. End-to-end operative repair of Achille tendon rupture. Am J Sports Med 1997;25:90–5.

8. Vosseller JT, Ellis SJ, Levine DS. Achilles tendon rupture in women. Foot Ankle Int 2013;34:49–53.

9. Nillius AS, Nilsson BE, Westlin NE. The incidence of Achilles tendon. Acta Orthop Scand 1976;47:118–21.

10. Moller A, Westlin NE. Increasing incidence of Achilles tendon rupture. Acta Orthop Scand 1996;67:479–81.

11. Leppilahti J, Puranen J, Orava S. Incidence of Achilles tendon rupture. Acta Orthop 1996;67:277–9.

12. Levi N. The incidence of Achilles tendon rupture in Copenhagen. Injury 1997;28:311–3.

13. Houshian S, Tscherning T, Riegels-Nielsen P. The epidemiology of Achilles tendon rupture in a Danish county. Injury 1998;29:651–4.

14. Maffulli N, Tallon C, Wong J, et al. Early weightbearing and ankle mobilization after open repair of acute midsubstance tears of the Achilles tendon. Am J Sports Med 2003;31:692–700.

15. Clayton RA, Court-Brown CM. The epidemiology of musculoskeletal tendinous and ligamentous injuries. Injury 2008;39:1338–44.

16. Jones BH, Bovee MW, Harris JM, et al. Intrinsic risk factors for exercise-related injuries among male and female army trainees. Am J Sports Med 1993;21:705–10.

17. Wojtys EM, Hust LJ, Lindenfeld TN, et al. Association between menstrual cycle and anterior cruciate ligament injuries in female athletes. Am J Sports Med 1998;26:614–9.

18. Wojtys EM, Huston LJ, Boynton MD. The effect of the menstrual cycle on anterior cruciate ligament injuries in women as determined by hormone levels. Am J Sports Med 2002;30:182–8.

19. Burgess KE, Pearson SJ, Onambele GL. Patellar tendon properties with fluctuating menstrual cycle hormones. J Strength Cond Res 2010;24:2088–95.

20. Burgess KE, Pearson SJ, Onambele GL. Menstrual cycle variations in oestradiol and progesterone have no impact on in vivo medial gastrocnemius tendon mechanical properties. Clin Biomech 2009;24:504–9.

21. Wentorf FA, Sudoh K, Moses C, et al. The effects of estrogen on material and mechanical properties of the intra- and extra-articular knee structures. Am J Sports Med 2006;34:1948–52.

22. Bryant AL, Clark RA, Bartold S, et al. Effects of estrogen on the mechanical behavior of the human Achilles tendon in vivo. J Appl Phys 2008;105:1035–43.

23. Kobori M, Yamamuro T. Effects of gonadectomy and estrogen administration on rat skeletal muscle. Clin Orthop 1989;243:306–11.

24. Jozsa L, Kvist M, Balint BJ, et al. The role of recreational sport activity in Achilles tendon rupture. A clinical, pathoanatomical, and sociological study of 292 cases. Am J Sports Med 1989;17:338–3434.

25. Davis JJ, Mason KT, Clark DA. Achilles tendon ruptures stratified by age, race, and cause of injury among active duty US military members. Mil Med 1999; 164:872–3.

26. Moller M, Movin T, Granhed H, et al. Acute rupture of tendon Achillis. A prospective randomised study of comparison between surgical and nonsurgical treatment. J Bone Joint Surg Br 2001;83:843–8.

27. Nilsson-Helander K, Silbernagel KG, Thomee R, et al. Acute Achilles tendon rupture: a randomized, controlled study comparing surgical and nonsurgical treatments using validated outcome measures. Am J Sports Med 2010;38: 2186–93.

28. Saleh M, Marshall PD, Senior R, et al. The Sheffield splint for controlled early mobilisation after rupture of the calcaneal tendon. A prospective, randomised comparison with plaster treatment. J Bone Joint Surg Br 1992;74:206–9.

29. Twaddle BC, Poon P. Early motion for Achilles tendon ruptures: is surgery important? A randomized, prospective study. Am J Sports Med 2007;35:2033–8.

30. Olsson N, Silbernagel KG, Eriksson BI, et al. Stable surgical repair with accelerated rehabilitation versus nonsurgical treatment for acute Achilles tendon ruptures: a randomized controlled study. Am J Sports Med 2013;41:2867–76.

31. De la Fuente C, Pena YLR, Carreno G, et al. Prospective randomized clinical trial of aggressive rehabilitation after acute Achilles tendon ruptures repaired with Dresden technique. Foot (Edinb) 2016;26:15–22.

32. Groetelaers RP, Janssen L, van der Velden J, et al. Functional treatment or cast immobilization after minimally invasive repair of an acute Achilles tendon rupture: prospective, randomized trial. Foot Ankle Int 2014;35:771–8.

33. Zhou K, Song L, Zhang P, et al. Surgical versus non-srugical methods for acute Achilles tendon rupture: a meta-analysis of randomized controlled trials. J Foot Ankle Surg 2018;57(6):1191–9.

34. Cetti R, Henriksen LO, Jacobsen KS. A new treatment of ruptured Achilles tendons. A prospective randomized study. Clin Orthop Relat Res 1994;308:155–65.

35. Manent A, Lopez L, Coromina H, et al. Acute Achilles tendon ruptures: efficacty of conservative and surgical (percutaneous, open) treatment – a randomized, controlled clinical trial. J Foot Ankle Surg 2019;58(6):1229–34.

36. Soroceanu A, Sidhwa F, Aarabi S, et al. Surgical versus nonsurgical treatment of acute Achilles tendon rupture: a meta-analysis of randomized trials. J Bone Joint Surg Am 2012;94:2136–43.

37. Watson TW, Jurist KA, Yang KH, et al. The strength of Achilles tendon repair: an in vitro study of the biomechanical behavior in human cadaver tendons. Foot Ankle Int 1995;16:191–5.

38. Jaakola JI, Hutton WC, Beskin JL, et al. Achilles tendon rupture repair: biomechanical comparison of the triple bundle technique versus the Krakow locking loop technique. Foot Ankle Int 2000;21:14–7.

39. Labib SA, Rolf R, Dacus R, et al. The "Giftbox" repair of the Achilles tendon: a modification of the Krackow technique. Foot Ankle Int 2009;30:410–4.

40. McCoy BW, Haddad SL. The strength of Achilles tendon repair: a comparison of three suture techniques in human cadaver tendons. Foot Ankle Int 2010;31: 701–5.

41. Backus JD, Marchetti DC, Slette EL, et al. Efficacy of suture caliber and number of core strands on repair of Achilles ruptures: a biomechanical study. Foot Ankle Int 2017;38:564–70.

42. Gnandt RJ, Smith JL, Nguyen-Ta K, et al. High-tensile strength tape versus high-tensile strength suture: a biomechanical study. Arthroscopy 2016;32:356–63.

43. Osei DA, Stepan JG, Calfee RP, et al. The effect of suture caliber and number of core suture strands on zone II flexor tendon repair: a study in human cadavers. J Hand Surg Am 2014;39:262–8.

44. Ma GWC, Griffith TG. Percutaneous repair of acute closed ruptured Achilles tendon: a new technique. Clin Orthop 1977;1128:247–55.

45. Clanton TO, Haytmanek CT, Williams BT, et al. A biomechanical comparison of an open repair and 3 minimally invasive percutaneous Achilles tendon repairs during a simulated progressive rehabilitation protocol. Am J Sports Med 2015;43: 1957–64.

46. Khan RJ, Fick D, Keogh A, et al. Treatment of acute Achilles tendon ruptures. A meta-analysis of randomized, controlled trials. J Bone Joint Surg Am 2005;87: 2202–10.

47. Bradley JP, Tibone JE. Percutaneous and open surgical repairs of Achilles tendon ruptures. A comparative study. Am J Sports Med 1990;18:188–95.

48. Assal M, Jung M, Stern R, et al. Limited open repair of Achilles tendon ruptures. A technique with a new instrument and findings of a prospective multicenter study. J Bone Joint Surg Am 2002;84:161–70.

49. Amlang MH, Christiani P, Heinz P, et al. Percutaneous technique for Achilles tedon repair with the Dresden instruments. Unfallchirurg 2005;108:529–36.

50. Hockenbury RT, Johns JC. A biomechanical in vitro comparison of open versus percutaneous repair of tendon Achilles. Foot Ankle 1990;11:67–72.

51. Haji A, Sahai A, Symes A, et al. Percutaneous versus open tendo Achillis repair. Foot Ankle Int 2004;25:215–8.

52. Lim J, Dalal R, Waseem M. Percutaneous vs. open repair of the ruptured Achilles tendon – a prospective randomized controlled study. Foot Ankle Int 2001;22: 559–68.

53. Cretnik A, Kosanovic M, Smrkolj V. Percutaneous versus open repair of the ruptured Achilles tendon: a comparative study. Am J Sports Med 2005;33: 1369–79.

54. Hsu AR, Jones CP, Cohen BE, et al. Clinical outcomes and complications of percutaneous Achilles repair system versus open techniques for acute Achilles tendon rupture. Foot Ankle Int 2015;36:1279–86.

55. Nistor L. Surgical and non-surgical treatment of Achilles tendon rupture. A prospective randomized study. J Bone Joint Surg Am 1981;63:394–9.

56. Cetti R, Christensen SE, Ejsted R, et al. Operative versus nonoperative treatment of Achilles tendon rupture. A prospective randomized study and review of the literature. Am J Sports Med 1993;21:791–9.

57. Bhandari M, Guyatt GH, Siddiqui F, et al. Treatment of acute Achilles tendon ruptures: a systematic overview and metaanalysis. Clin Orthop Relat Res 2002;400: 190–200.

58. Erickson BJ, Mascarenhas R, Saltzman BM, et al. Is operative treatment of Achilles tendon ruptures superior to nonoperative treatment? A systematic review of overlapping meta-analyses. Orthop J Sports Med 2015;3(suppl 2):1–6.

59. Jones MP, Khan RJK, Carey RL. Surgical interventions for treating acute Achilles tendon rupture: key findings from a recent Cochrane review. J Bone Joint Surg Am 2012;94:e88.

60. Jacob K, Paterson R. Surgical repair followed by functional rehabilitation for acute and chronic Achilles tendon injuries: excellent functional results, patient satisfaction and no reruptures. ANZ J Surg 2007;77:287–91.

61. Metz R, Verleisdonk EJ, van der Heijden, et al. Acute Achilles tendon rupture: minimally invasive surgery versus nonoperative treatment with immediate full weight-bearing – a randomized controlled trial. Am J Sports Med 2008;36: 1688–94.

62. Lantto I, Hiekkinen J, Flinkkila T, et al. A prospective randomized trial comparing surgical and nonsurgical treatments of acute Achilles tendon ruptures. Am J Sports Med 2016;44:2406–14.

63. Willits K, Amendola A, Bryant D, et al. Operative versus nonoperative treatment of acute Achilles tendon ruptures: a multicenter randomized trial using accelerated functional rehabilitation. J Bone Joint Surg Am 2010;92:2767–75.

64. Manent A, Lopez L, Vilanova J, et al. Assessment of the resistance of several suture techniques in human cadaver Achilles tendons. J Foot Ankle Surg 2017;56: 954–9.

65. Deng S, Sun Z, Zhang C, et al. Surgical treatment versus conservative management for acute Achilles tendon rupture: s systemic review and meta-analysis of randomized controlled trials. J Foot Ankle Surg 2017;56:1236–43.

66. Cottom JM, Baker JS, Richardson PE, et al. Evaluation of a new knotless suture anchor repair in acute Achilles tendon ruptures: a biomechanical comparison of three techniques. J Foot Ankle Surg 2017;56:423–7.

67. Demetracopoulos CA, Gilbert SL, Young E, et al. Limited-open Achilles tendon repair using locking sutures versus nonlocking sutures: an in vitro model. Foot Ankle Int 2014;35:612–8.

68. Grassi A, Annunziato A, Kristian S, et al. Minimally invasive versus open repair for acute Achilles tendon rupture. J Bone Joint Surg Am 2018;100:1969–81.

69. Cretnik A, Kosanovic M, Kosir R. Long-term results with the use of modified percutaneous repair of the ruptured Achilles tendon under local anaesthesia. J Foot Ankle Surg 2019;58:828–36.

70. Lansdaal JR, Goslings JC, Reichart M, et al. The results of 163 Achilles tendon ruptures treated by a minimally invasive surgical technique and functional aftertreatment. Injury 2007;38:839–44.

71. Majewski M, Rohrbach M, Czaja S, et al. Avoiding sural nerve injuries during percutaneous Achilles tendon repair. Am J Sports Med 2006;34:793–8.

72. McMahon SE, Smith TO, Hing CB. A meta-analysis of randomized controlled trials comparing conventional to minimally invasive approaches for repair of an Achilles tendon rupture. Foot Ankle Surg 2011;17:211–7.

73. Rozis M, Benetos I, Karampinas P, et al. Outcome of percutaneous fixation of acute Achilles tendon ruptures. Foot Ankle Int 2018;39:689–93.

74. Yang B, Liu Y, Kan S, et al. Outcomes and complications of percutaneous versus open repair of acute Achilles tendon rupture: a meta-analysis. Int J Surg 2017;40: 178–86.

75. Wilkins R, Bisson LJ. Operative versus nonoperative management of acute Achilles tendon ruptures: a quantitative systemic review of randomized controlled trials. Am J Sports Med 2012;40:2154–60.

76. Cretnik A, Kosanovic M, Smrkolj V. Percutaneous suturing of the ruptured Achilles tendon under local anesthesia. J Foot Ankle Surg 2004;43:72–81.

77. Shepull T, Kvist J, Norman H, et al. Autologous platelets have no effect on the healing of human Achilles tendon ruptures. Am J Sports Med 2011;39:38–47.

78. Ollivere BJ, Bosman HA, Bearcroft PW, et al. Foreign body granulomatous reaction associated with polyethelene 'Fiberwire(®)' suture material used in Achilles tendon repair. Foot Ankle Surg 2014;20:e27–9.

79. de Cesar Netto C, Bernasconi A, Roberts L, et al. Open re-rupture of the Achilles tendon following minimally invasive repair: a case report. J Foot Ankle Surg 2018; 57:1272–7.

80. Healy B, Beasley R, Weatherall M. Venous thromboembolism following prolonged cast immobilisation for injury to the tendo Achillis. J Bone Joint Surg Br 2010;92: 646–50.

81. Calder JDF, Freeman R, Domeij-Arverud E, et al. Metaanalysis and suggested guidelines for prevention of venous thromboembolism (VTE) in foot and ankle surgery. Knee Surg Sports Traumatol Arthrosc 2016;24:1409–20.

82. Patel A, Ogawa B, Charlton T, et al. Incidence of deep vein thrombosis and pulmonary embolism after Achilles tendon rupture. Clin Orthop Relat Res 2012;470: 270–4.

Calcaneal Bone Tumors

Eric W. Temple, DPM[a,b,]*, Ryan D. Prusa, DPM, PGY2[a,b]

KEYWORDS

• Calcaneus • Bone • Tumor • Surgical • Benign • Malignant • Lesion

KEY POINTS

- Calcaneal bone tumors are an uncommon finding in the calcaneus but must be part of the provider's differential diagnosis.
- Clinical presentation can involve pain and swelling when symptomatic, but most benign lesions are discovered incidentally on imaging.
- Imaging plays a key role in the identification of lesions with discovery typically occurring with plain film radiographs, and more advanced imaging can be helpful for diagnosis.
- Treatment typically involves curettage and possible bone grafting for benign lesions and more aggressive resection or amputation for malignant lesions.

INTRODUCTION

Bone tumors of the foot are an uncommon finding with only around 3% of all skeletal tumors.[1] Of these foot tumors most are benign and outnumber the malignant lesions by at least 4 to 1.[2] Consequently, the diagnosis of malignant tumors can be delayed due to the practitioner assuming a tumor may be benign.[1] Often misdiagnosed as soft tissue injuries due to their rare presentation in the foot and ankle, the practitioner must remember to consider bone tumors in their differential.[3] The history and physical examination play an important role in diagnosis. Pain will often be a presenting complaint.[4] Special attention should be paid to the duration, quality, course, and onset of pain. Effectiveness of treatments tried by the patient should also be considered as factors relating to when the patient's pain is worst and if certain medications such as aspirin provide relief can help with narrowing a diagnosis.

Imaging plays an important role, and most tumors can at least be initially seen with plain film radiographs. Incidental discovery of calcaneal lesions also commonly occurs due to many lesions being asymptomatic.[5] Classification with plain films can be difficult, and advanced imaging such as computed tomography (CT) or MRI may need to be obtained. No matter what imaging modality is being used, all tumors should be characterized using a standard set of important information. The description will include the site, size, density, margin characteristics, and effect on natural cortical barrier of the bone.[2]

[a] The Iowa Clinic, 5950 University Avenue West, Des Moines, IA 50266, USA; [b] Unitypoint Health - Iowa Methodist Medical Center, 1415 Woodland Avenue, Des Moines, IA 50309, USA
* Corresponding author. The Iowa Clinic, 5950 University Avenue West, Des Moines, IA 50266.
E-mail address: etemple@iowaclinic.com

Clin Podiatr Med Surg 38 (2021) 227–233
https://doi.org/10.1016/j.cpm.2020.12.007
0891-8422/21/© 2021 Elsevier Inc. All rights reserved.

Treatments are variable, and it can be expected that patients with benign lesions will have good outcomes, whereas those with malignant lesions are likely to result in the necessity for more aggressive surgery and thus increased disability.[6] Benign symptomatic lesions can typically be treated with curettage and grafting.[5]

This writing provides a brief overview of each of the bone tumors that are known to present in the calcaneus.

DISCUSSION
Benign Lesions

Unicameral bone cyst

The calcaneus accounts for approximately 75% to 85% of all unicameral bone cysts found in the foot.[2] These lesions begin early in life as children and begin to enlarge once the patient has reached skeletal maturity. Typically, the lesions are asymptomatic and discovered incidentally on radiographs. A 2 cm to 3 cm radiolucent area with sclerotic margins will be seen on radiograph.[7] The lesions typically do not expand or violate cortical margins. The natural structure of the bone can be weakened, and although rare, pathologic fracture is possible.[6]

Treatment is indicated if pathologic fracture occurs or is highly likely to occur and if pain is present.[8] The most common treatment includes curettage, irrigation, and packing of the lesion with bone graft. The graft can be either autogenous or allogenic based on the surgeon's preference. Intraoperatively the lesion is described as a serous fluid-filled cavity with striplike bony prominences and a thin fibrous membrane.[6] Patients who do require surgery typically heal well with a low rate of recurrence.

Aneurysmal bone cyst

Aneurysmal bone cysts are benign locally aggressive tumors that account for 1% to 2% of primary bone tumors.[9] Unlike unicameral bone cysts patients with aneurysmal bone cysts will often present with a palpable tender mass. The patient can present with heel pain after minor trauma or pain while walking. They typically are found in the tarsals and metatarsals, but it is possible for them to occur in the calcaneus. Plain film radiographs will show some distinct features that will help in identification. There will be bulging of the cortex and trabeculation or honeycombing inside the lesion itself.[2]

The aneurysmal bone cyst will contain hemorrhagic fluid when aspirated or opened. Surgical intervention with debridement, irrigation, and bone grafting is the treatment of choice. Local recurrence when only curettage is performed is reported to be around 31% and will commonly cause destruction of surrounding joints that can lead to functional deficits.[9] Adjuvant therapy can be used, and recurrence rates are dropped to between 3.7% and 18%.[9] These include cryotherapy, phenol, polymethylmethacrylate, and radiation.[6]

Osteoid osteoma/osteoblastoma

Only differing in size, osteoid osteoma and osteoblastoma are a benign bone lesion that typically present in the tarsal bones. Osteoid osteoma is a lesion that is less than 2 cm, whereas an osteoblastoma is greater than 2 cm. Typically, these lesions are present in patients who are in the second and third decades of life. Incidence is higher in the male population with around 75% of cases.[6] Pain is present with a slow gradual onset over time, and symptoms are worse in the evenings. Diagnostically the lesion is unique in that pain can be relieved with aspirin.

On plain radiographs the tumor will be radiolucency in the periphery and either radiolucency or calcification centrally. If the lesion is in its early stages, it might be difficult to visualize on plain films and will be able to be seen more apparently on CT or MRI. CT scan will demonstrate a well-defined nidus with a smoothly margined lytic lesion with central mineralization. Although symptom management can be undertaken with aspirin in the nonsurgical candidate, resection with curettage is the most common treatment.

Osteochondroma
Rarely seen in the calcaneus, 10% of osteochondromas of the foot and hand are found in the heel.[6] The lesion is only found in patients younger than 20 years implying a malignant transformation in adults. Patients present initially with a painless enlarging mass. A presentation of pain will be related to pathologic fractures or malignant transformation. Physical examination will reveal a firm, nonmobile painful nodular mass.

Radiographic imaging will reveal a solitary bone prominence that is pedunculated or sessile.[6] Although a hyaline cartilage cap is present on the lesion, it will not be able to be visualized on radiograph. CT imaging will show the cartilage cap and is also useful to reveal the true size of the lesion. Malignant transformation to chondrosarcoma can be differentiated by a cartilage cap with a thickness of greater than 1.5 cm.[6] The most accurate way to measure the cartilage cap is by MRI. Asymptomatic lesions typically do not require treatment. Surgical excision with adequate margins should be undertaken when the lesion has transformed to a malignant classification. When complete excision is undertaken reoccurrence is low.[6]

Chondroblastoma
Chondroblastomas are a benign cartilaginous neoplasm of bone that will most frequently appear in the calcaneus or the talus when found in the foot. They make up around 1% to 2% of all primary bone tumors.[10] The lesion will arise from an active epiphyseal plate in a patient who is between 10 to 20 years of age.[2] A male predominance ratio of 5:1 is observed.[6] Local pain and swelling can be presenting symptoms, although asymptomatic lesions can also be found incidentally on radiographs.[11]

On radiographs the lesion will be radiolucent with sclerotic margins or tiny stippled calcifications. If MRI is obtained it will reveal an irregular, expansive lesion and fluid-filled levels.[11] Histologically the lesion will have rich glycogen granules separated by cartilaginous matrix in histiocytic cells.[10] Immunostaining will be helpful in diagnosis as well. Treatment is commonly done surgically with curettage and grafting. Primary arthrodesis or even calcanectomy might be necessary depending on the size and location of the tumor.[3] Recurrence is not uncommon, and adjuvant therapies such as cautery or cryotherapy can be used to reduce this risk.[3]

Giant cell tumor of bone
Giant cell tumors are not commonly found in the foot, with approximately 2% of all occurrences being found in the foot.[2] When in the foot they are typically in the calcaneus and metatarsals. Men are affected 3 times more than women.[2] Clinical presentation typically involves heel pain and swelling.

Radiographically the tumors are radiolucent with a small peripheral zone of sclerosis. Histologically the tumor is made up of numerous multinucleated giant cells. Treatment is typically curettage. Giant cell tumors can be very aggressive in nature, and additional adjuvant treatments are recommended. Intralesional cryotherapy, phenol, polymethylmethacrylate, or cauterization can be used. Even with these extra steps recurrence is between 10% and 30%. Patients should be educated on the possibility of recurrence and the need for possible future wide excision requiring reconstruction or even amputation.

Intraosseous lipoma

Intraosseous lipomas are a rare tumor reported to make up only 0.1% of all bone tumors.[8] Of these, only 8% are located in the calcaneus.[6] However, incidence is on the increase with the widespread use of diagnostic imaging.[12] The tumors themselves are often asymptomatic and identified incidentally. When a patient does experience symptoms, they are commonly local pain and edema that could easily be misdiagnosed as more common presenting conditions such as plantar fasciitis or retrocalcaneal bursitis.[13] Pathologic fracture is rare but can occur.

Radiographically the lesion is well defined but expansile. Cortical thinning is possible, and marginal sclerosis is typically not present. Histologically the tumor is composed of fat cells surrounded by necrosis and calcification along with areas of hemorrhage and bony trabeculae.[6] Asymptomatic tumors that are in nonweight-bearing areas can be treated conservatively. For patients at high risk for or have a pathologic fracture, curettage and packing with bone graft is the treatment of choice. Internal fixation may also be indicated for fracture or if high risk of fracture after curettage is identified.[12,13] Low recurrence and complications are reported.[6]

In a study by Toepfer and colleagues in 2016 endoscopic resection and allografting was used. Two portals were established into the calcaneus, and a shaver was used to remove the lipoma. The space was then packed with allogenic cancellous bone chips. Their case series included 3 patients. Thy reported a success rate of 100%, and all patients had returned to everyday activities in normal shoe gear 6 weeks after surgery.[8]

Ganglion of bone

Intraosseous ganglions are most commonly found in the calcaneus and cuboid. Overall, their occurrence is extremely rare. Plain radiographs reveal epiphyseal or metaphyseal location with a round of oval lytic area, which could be uniocular or multilocular. No periosteal reaction or cortical changes are typically noted. Treatment again involved curettage and packing of the lesion with bone graft. Intraoperatively the fluid from within the tumor will be consistent with the straw-colored fluid of any other ganglion cyst. Attempt should be made to find the capsule of the cyst and completely remove it.

Enchondroma

Enchondroma is a cartilaginous tumor that will typically be present in patients between the second and sixth decades of life. Intermittent pain and swelling are possible. The most commonly affected areas in the foot are the phalanges and metatarsals, but it is possible for an enchondroma to be present in the calcaneus. Pathologic fracture is the primary concern with this lesion.

The tumor will radiate from the medullary area with possible cortical expansion and thinning. Treatment is curettage and bone grafting. Complete removal of the lesion is important, as recurrence is a concern.

Malignant Lesions

Ewing sarcoma

Ewing sarcoma is the most common primary malignant tumor of bone in the foot. More than 50% of cases occur in the foot.[6] The most common location in the foot is the calcaneus and is associated with high mortality rates. Typically, patients will be between 5 and 15 years old. Pain and swelling are common presenting complaints. Constitutional symptoms of fever and weight loss can also be observed. On physical examination, stretched and shiny skin with dilated subcutaneous veins will be present due to extensive swelling around the heel. Laboratory testing can be helpful in diagnosis with elevated erythrocyte sedimentation rate (ESR), acid phosphatase, and white blood cells. Moderate anemia is commonly seen as well.

Radiographically the tumor will show permeation and commonly expansion. This destruction is commonly referred to as a "moth-eaten" appearance. Because of the high mortality associated with Ewing sarcoma, oncology consult is recommended before any biopsy or treatment is performed. Metastasis is high and commonly found in the lungs and other bones. Chemotherapy, radiation, and amputation are common treatments.

Osteogenic sarcoma

Although this tumor is the most common nonhaemopoietic primary malignant neoplasm of bone, osteogenic sarcoma is exceedingly rare in the foot and even more rare in the calcaneus, as the tumor is typically seen in the metatarsals. Clinical presentation often involves worsening pain and swelling of the adjacent ankle joint. The tumor is extremely aggressive and is able to be identified radiographically by invasion into adjacent soft tissue and evidence of rapid bony destruction and proliferation. ESR and C-reactive protein will be elevated on laboratory testing. Metastasis occurs early and often. Treatment includes aggressive excision or amputation with close follow-up. Chemotherapy is commonly needed as well.

Chondrosarcoma

Chondrosarcomas are rarely seen in the foot. When seen they are most commonly found in the calcaneus, phalanges, and metatarsals. Clinical presentation includes an insidious gradual onset of pain. Radiographically the tumor will be expansile with cortical destruction and expansion into the soft tissues. MRI is typically indicated, as it is able to help determine the extent of the lesion. A well lobulated mass with high signal intensity of the T2-weighted image is observed due to the high water content of the cartilage-based tumor. Treatment can vary depending on the size and location of the lesion, but prognosis is better than other malignant bone tumors. Wide surgical resection or amputation are top treatment choices, with amputation being performed in up to half of cases.[1] Local excision or curettage is not effective due to high recurrence rates.

Metastatic lesions

Metastatic lesions are rarely seen in the foot, but when present the calcaneus is the most common location they are seen.[14] Most common primary sites of tumors that metastasized to the foot include breast, bladder, lung, kidney, and colorectal. Treatments for these lesions can vary widely based on prognosis of the patient and can range from curettage to below knee amputation.[3] When involved, the foot and ankle surgeon will be part of a multidisciplinary team taking care of the patient.

SUMMARY

Calcaneal bone tumors can represent a challenging component to the foot and ankle surgeon. Because of the rarity of these lesions they are not commonly encountered during practice, and delay in diagnosis is not unusual.[3] When they occur, it is important to use all available diagnostic testing and imaging to aide in their identification. With many lesions found incidentally on imaging it is critical for the physician to be able to differentiate between benign tumors and malignant ones; this can be particularly challenging due to the lack of reliable diagnostic signs from the physical examination or history.[14] Malignant and benign lesions cannot be determined by pain, lesion size, and symptom duration.[1] Imaging will play a key role in diagnosis, and CT and MRI should be obtained. Biopsy can be performed, and histologic analysis is key for definitive diagnosis. The most common treatment of benign lesions is curettage and grafting. Wide excision or amputation must be considered for malignant tumors to prevent metastasis. The foot and ankle surgeon must have a solid understanding of these tumors, so when encountered appropriate treatment can be performed.

CLINICS CARE POINTS

- Calcaneal bone tumors are an uncommon finding in the calcaneus but must be part of the provider's differential diagnosis.
- Clinical presentation can involve pain and swelling when symptomatic, but most benign lesions are discovered incidentally on imaging.
- Imaging will play a key role in identification of lesions with discovery typically occurring with plain film radiographs, and more advanced imaging can be helpful for diagnosis.
- Treatment typically involves curettage and possible bone grafting for benign lesions and more aggressive resection or amputation for malignant lesions.

DISCLOSURE

The authors have nothing to disclose.

REFERENCES

1. Ruggieri P, Angelini A, Jorge FD, et al. Review of foot tumors seen in a university tumor institute. J Foot Ankle Surg 2014;53(3):282–5.
2. McGlamry M. Lesions of the heel. The Podiatry Institute Update; 1997. p. 213–9. Chapter 35.
3. Young PS, Bell SW, MacDuff EM, et al. Primary osseous tumors of the hindfoot: why the delay in diagnosis and should we be concerned? Clin Orthop Relat Res 2013;471(3):871–7.
4. Berlin SJ, Mirkin GS, Tubridy SP. Tumors of the heel. Clin Podiatr Med Surg 1990; 7(2):307–21.
5. Oommen AT, Madhuri V, Walter NM. Benign tumors and tumor-like lesions of the calcaneum: a study of 12 cases. Indian J Cancer 2009;46(3):234–6.
6. Yan L, Zong J, Chu J, et al. Primary tumours of the calcaneus. Oncol Lett 2018; 15(6):8901–14.
7. Malghem J, Lecouvet F, Vande Berg B. Calcaneal cysts and lipomas: a common pathogenesis? Skeletal Radiol 2017;46(12):1635–42.
8. Toepfer A, Lenze U, Gerdesmeyer L, et al. Endoscopic resection and allografting for benign osteolytic lesions of the calcaneus. Springerplus 2016;5:427.
9. Bosco ALD, Nunes MC, Kim JH, et al. Hindfoot aneurysmal bone cyst: report of two cases. Rev Bras Ortop 2018;53(2):257–65.
10. Chen J, Jie K, Feng W, et al. Total calcanectomy and bilateral iliac bone autograft reconstruction for the treatment of calcaneal chondroblastoma involving a secondary aneurysmal bone cyst: a case report and literature review. J Foot Ankle Surg 2020;59(3):616–24.
11. Blitch E, Mendicino RW. Chondroblastoma of the calcaneus: literature review and case presentation. J Foot Ankle Surg 1996;35(3):250–4.

12. Frangež I, Nizič-Kos T, Cimerman M. Threatening fracture of intraosseous lipoma treated by internal fixation case report and review of the literature. J Am Podiatr Med Assoc 2019;109(1):75–9.
13. Azarsina S, Biglari F, Hassanmirzaei B, et al. Intraosseous lipoma of calcaneus, rare cause of chronic calcaneal pain: a case report. Arch Bone Jt Surg 2019; 7(5):469–73.
14. Chou LB, Ho YY, Malawer MM. Tumors of the foot and ankle: experience with 153 cases. Foot Ankle Int 2009;30(9):836–41.

Biologics in the Treatment of Achilles Tendon

William T. DeCarbo, DPM*

KEYWORDS

• Achilles • Tendinitis • Biologics • Stems cells • Platelet rich plasma

KEY POINTS

- Minimally invasive or surgical treatment of Achilles tendinitis using biologics.
- The use of biologics to augment the surgical treatment of Achilles tendinitis.
- The published outcomes of the use of biologics in Achilles tendinitis treatment.

INTRODUCTION

Pathologies of the Achilles tendon are either due to acute injuries, usually sport related, or chronic in nature, which are referred to as Achilles tendinopathies. Achilles tendinopathy leads to a repetitive microtrauma, which is caused by an overload stress or overuse.[1] This microtrauma leads to pain, swelling, and lack of function of the Achilles tendon. This group of symptoms is said to be a result of the failed response of the tendon to heal.[2] This tendinopathy is characterized by an excessive proliferation of tenocytes and a change in their morphology, the disruption of collagen fibers, and increase in glycosaminoglycans, which is a noncollagenous matrix, fat tissue, and neovascularization.[3–5] The question remains that with this lack to cellular response with Achilles tendon pathology can the healing response be accelerated or improved with the use of biological augmentation?

Typical Achilles tendinitis can be successfully treated with conservative treatment including rest, immobilization, antiinflammatories, stretching, activity modification, and physical therapy in the acute setting. If initial treatment is unsuccessful, a transformation to a more chronic condition or even Achilles tendinosis may occur. This is primarily due to the inability of the Achilles tendon to heal itself attributed to the hypocellularity and hypovascularity of the tendon.[6] Both the acute and chronic conditions usually affect the midsubstance of the Achilles, which is 2 cm to 6 cm from the posterior insertion site. This acute and chronic pathology can also affect the insertion of the Achilles tendon. This pathology often leads to a mechanically weak tissue composed of a fibrovascular scar[7] The fibrovascular scar tissue poses a risk of future reinjury, recurrence, or possible rupture due to this weakening.[8]

St. Clair Orthopedic Associates, 1050 Bower Hill Road, Suite 105, Pittsburgh, PA 14243, USA
* 1768 Sapphire Court, Pittsburgh, PA 15241.
E-mail address: wdecarbo@yahoo.com

Clin Podiatr Med Surg 38 (2021) 235–244
https://doi.org/10.1016/j.cpm.2020.12.008
0891-8422/21/© 2021 Elsevier Inc. All rights reserved.

podiatric.theclinics.com

When the abovementioned conservative treatment fails, patients are often left with surgical options that typically involve prolonged recovery with limited weight bearing. Biologics present an augment to healing that may limit surgical exposure and hasten recovery times. The biological augmentation for the Achilles tendon may improve the tendon quality biomechanically and enhance the healing process.[9]

To date, several biologics to help improve outcomes have been reported on. These include platelet-rich plasma (PRP), bone marrow aspirate concentrate (BMAC), growth factors, adipose-derived stem cell (ADSCs), peripheral blood mononuclear cells (PBMNCs), and scaffolds for both cellular growth and structural support.[10]

DISCUSSION

PRP contains concentrated platelets from blood, which contains mostly white blood cells. PRP is thought to be safe due to the autologous nature of this biologic. PRP contains many growth factors, including platelet-derived growth factors (PDGF), transforming growth factor beta (TGF-B), vascular endothelial growth factor (VEGF), and hepatocytes, which potentially enhance tendon healing while providing a scaffold for the cells (**Fig. 1**).

A classification system proposed by Dohan Ehrenfest and colleagues[11] separates the different PRP preparation into 4 main cellular make-ups, which include pure PRP (leukocyte-poor PRP), leukocyte and PRP, pure platelet-rich fibrin (leukocyte-poor platelet-rich fibrin), and leukocyte and platelet-rich fibrin.

Pure PRP, also known as leukocyte-poor PRP, is composed of a low-density fibrin network without leukocytes. This preparation can be used as either a liquid or a gel in its activated form.

Leukocyte and PRP contains both leukocytes and low-density fibrin in its activated form. This preparation is most common with the many commercially available systems on the market.

Pure platelet-rich fibrin, also known as leukocyte-poor platelet-rich fibrin, is a mixture without leukocytes but with a high-density fibrin network. This preparation when activated is in gel form only and as such cannot be injected. This preparation is also very costly when compared with other platelet-rich fibrin products.

Lastly, leukocyte and platelet-rich fibrin are products with leukocytes and high-density fibrin. This preparation also is in gel form only, hence cannot be injected; however, it can be handled as a solid.

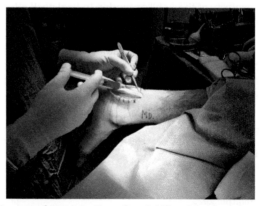

Fig. 1. Intraoperative use of PRP injection after Achilles debridement.

When using PRP for the treatment of both Achilles tendinitis or tendinosis that has failed conservative efforts, the efficacy and improvement of outcome remains a topic of debate. Lin and colleagues[12] did a meta-analysis that identified 7 articles comparing the use of autologous blood-derived products versus a placebo, which was either sham injection, no injection, or physical therapy alone in patients with Achilles pathology. The results revealed equivocal outcomes between the 2 groups in the Victorian Institute of Sports Assessment-Achilles questionnaire (VISA-A) score improvements with assessments made at 4 to 6 weeks, 6 weeks, 12 weeks, 24 weeks, and 48 weeks. There was also no change between VISA-A scores at the short-, medium-, or long-term intervals (4–6 weeks, 12 weeks, and 24 weeks, respectively). The results of this study showed no improved effectiveness between the PRP and placebo groups and no improvement in symptom duration.

The results of the paper noted earlier encompass more chronic Achilles conditions. Although outside the scope of this article, PRP augmentations have also been looked at in the more acute setting of Achilles ruptures. A review by Filardo and colleagues[13] looked at the application of PRP in the Achilles rupture when it was repaired by suture. This review again yielded no measurable benefits of PRP effecting the Achilles repair or outcome.

BMAC, which concentrates the mononucleated cells, hematopoietic stem cells, and platelets in one layer and red blood cells in another layer, has also been used in Achilles pathology (**Fig. 2**). The idea behind the use of BMAC is to control inflammation, reduce fibrosis, and recruit tenocytes and mesenchymal stem cells to the damaged tendon tissue.[14] The use of BMAC has not been reported in the chronic Achilles condition; however, one study looked at its use again in the acute setting.[15] Achilles tendon ruptures of 27 patients were augmented with BMAC, of which 92% returned to sport at 5.9 ± 1.8 months with no reruptures noted.

Growth factors and PDGF are also biological options to augment Achilles tendon pathology. Growth factors in general are involved in the activation and regulation of the cellular response when a tendon is injured.[16] This cellular response is involved in the proliferation and synthesis of extracellular matrix and differentiation of cell chemotaxis. These cells, which are produced by tenocytes and white blood cells, are released from the platelets during a process called degranulation.[16]

TGF-B is composed of 3 different protein isoforms including TGF-B1, B2, and B3. TGF-B1 is overexpressed early in the injury process.[17] TGF-B is released at too high levels leading to destabilization of the extracellular matrix resulting in tenocyte death.[18] According to in vivo and in vitro studies, if TGF-B1 can be stopped this possibly leads to a decrease in tendon adhesions, which results in an increase in the tendon's range of motion.[19,20] Therefore, TGF-B therapy has the potential to

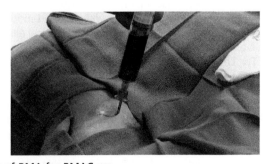

Fig. 2. Harvesting of BMA for BMAC use.

influence Achilles tendon healing by increasing the mechanical strength by the regulation of collagen synthesis, enhanced matrix remodeling, and the upregulation of cross-link formations.[21]

VEGF is also a family of isoforms consisting of VEGF-A, B, C, D, E, and placenta growth factor. VEGF-A has been shown present with excessive scar tissue formation due to its neovascularization for tissue healing.[22] This increase in VEGF has been shown most prevalent in the 7- to 10-day period of tendon repair, peaking at day 14, suggesting the repair site is undergoing neovascularization.[23] In an attempt to demonstrate the role of VEGF-A, Temper and colleagues (1:44) blocked its signal with a monoclonal antibody, Bevacizumab, in rats with complete Achilles ruptures. The result was a significant decrease in angiogenesis, which led to reduced cross-sectional area of the tendon, improved matrix organization, increased stiffness, and a reduction of maximum load and stress.[24]

PDGF is a protein also existing in 3 isoforms: PDGF-AA, PDGF-BB, and PDGF-AB. These isoforms help to increase type I collagen by acting as chemotactic agents.[25] Exogenous PDGF increase tenocyte expression of type I collagen.[26] This increase in PDGF and specifically PDGF-BB has been shown to improve tendon function.[27,28]

Insulin-like growth factor (IGF) is a family of single-chain polypeptides, which include IGF-I, IGF-II, and insulin. IGF-I has been shown to have a positive effect on tendon healing on transected rat Achilles tendons.[29] Furthermore, IGF-I with the addition of PRP increased expression throughout the healing process of both epitenon and endotenon in Achilles tendon ruptures.[29]

PBMNCs are composed of monocytes, macrophages, and lymphocytes. PBMNCs are thought to be a new generation of regenerative autologous cell concentrates that guide regeneration and promote the repair of tissue.[30–32] The advantage of BMA with pluripotent stem cells is the ability to differentiate into other cells. The same can be said for monocytes and macrophages. They have been shown to differentiate into their surrounding tissues microenvironment and also increase the release of VEGF, which facilitates the angiogenic action.[33–36]

Scaffold to promote mechanical support and cellular growth in Achilles tendon repair have been described more recently. Scaffold is composed of both natural and synthetic materials including collagen, silk, polymers, and hybrid materials.[10] Scaffold acts to release and recruit chemotactic factors and progenitor cells,[37] which ideally allows a bridging of a tendinous defect with ultimately a complete incorporation of the material into the tendon. Decellularized tendon tissue is often used with tendon augmentation to act as scaffold. The advantage of decellularized tendon tissue is the preservation of proteoglycans and growth factors and maintenance of tensile strength of the extracellular matrix, ultrastructure, and biochemical composition.[38] Farnebo and colleagues[39] have demonstrated an enhancement of mechanical properties all while reducing the immune response in rats using decellularized grafts. Porcine tendon has also been shown to be recellularized with human tenocytes.[40] In contrast to decellularized are acellular grafts composed of human dermal allograft. This graft is a commercially available product by the name GraftJacket (Wright medical Technology, Inc, Arlington, TN, USA). Studies in vivo showed an increase in return to activity in patients without complication reported with this biologic.[41,42]

Xenografts have also been described as scaffolds, specifically the small intestinal submucosa of porcine.[43] Small intestine submucosa retains several biologically active growth factors (VEGF, TGF-B, and fibroblasts) that attract cell migration into the graft.[44,45] The positive about the use of small intestine submucosa graft is its ability for rapid and complete degradation. Sixty percent of the graft is lost in the first 30 days with complete degradation within 90 days, and this allows the extracellular matrix of the tendon to look similar to native tissue in regard to the vascularity and organization of the tissue.[44] An additional positive when using small intestine submucosa graft is the ability to recruit marrow-derived cells during the repair and remodeling process.[45]

The scaffolds can be used as on-lay grafts, interpositioned within the tendon or circumferentially wrapped around the tendon (**Figs. 3** and **4**).

Imaging is an important discussion point when determining Achilles tendon pathology and the augmentation of biologics. The involvement of the damaged tendon and the specific area of damage can be assessed with MRI, which is probably the most common modality used, ultrasonography, and sonoelastography.

MRI is widely used in Achilles tendon pathology and has several advantages. MRI is not user dependent as ultrasound and sonoelastography. MRI technology can differentiate between paratenonitis and tendinosis and determine the extent of degeneration of the tendon along with exact location of the damage. This exact extent and location of pathology is useful for the surgical planning and potential biological use for patients. MRI is also useful postsurgical procedure and biological use to assess the effects of treatment.

Oloff and colleagues[46] created a classification system that is composed of 5 grades based on the thickness and signal changes of the tendon. The grades range from hypertrophy to severe thickness, and the signal changes range from homogeneous to greater than 50% abnormal tendon signal or partial tendon tear. Fildardo and colleagues[13] reviewed 13 patients who were treated for Achilles debridement with application of PRP and 13 patients who were treated with PRP alone. Pretreatment and posttreatment clinical outcomes were assessed. In conclusion, the Pearson's

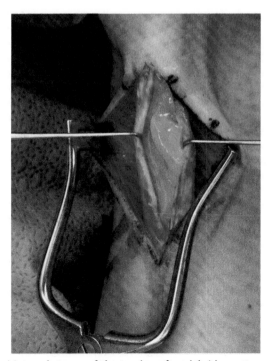

Fig. 3. Graft placed intrasubstance of the tendon after debridement.

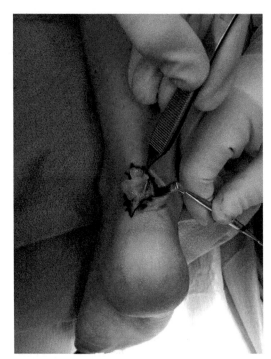

Fig. 4. On-lay graft after debridement of the tendon.

correlation test showed a linear pattern between the difference in MRI score and VISA-A score where the VISA-A score alone did not correlate with the MRI score.

Albano and colleagues[47] also assessed posttreatment changes using MRI with Achilles treated with either ADSCs or PRP. Both treatments showed an increase in the tendon thickness via MRI posttreatment.

Ultrasonography technology has been described for diagnosis of Achilles tendon pathology, which can determine tendinosis, partial or complete Achilles tendon ruptures, and the extend to tissue damage. The Achilles tendon has several advantages that make ultrasound use a good choice. The Achilles tendon is easily accessible in the posterior leg, has a large volume of tissue to assess, is straight from its origin to insertion, and allows for a dynamic evaluation with both active and passive Achilles tendon range of motion.[48] Also, ultrasound has the capability to, in theory, demonstrate hyperemia, increased vascularity, and varicosities with the use of color doppler imaging[49] (**Fig. 5**).

Albano and colleagues[47] performed intratendinous leucocyte-rich PRP or ADSCs injections into the Achilles tendon for noninsertion Achilles pathology patients. They assess the correlation between ultrasound and clinical outcomes. What was shown was a significant increase in tendon thickness postinjection, but no significant difference was noted in cross-section area of the tendon, signal intensity, or echotexture when comparing the pre- and posttreatment ultrasound scans.

Sonoelastography is another imaging modality that is ultrasound based. This modality analyzes the tissue as a deforming force by the examiner is applied. What is analyzed is the viscoelastic behavior of the tissue being examined.[50] This technology works by using real-time Doppler ultrasound, which creates images from the vibration created by low-frequency waves through the tissue being examined. This image is returned as a scale of colors that range from blue to green and yellow to red: blue

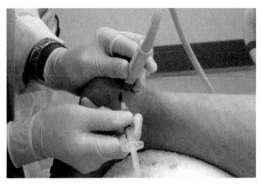

Fig. 5. Ultrasound-guided biological Achilles injection.

indicates maximum stiffness, green and yellow indicate intermediate stiffness, and red indicates the greatest elasticity.[50] Sonoelastography is used clinically in those patients with a symptomatic Achilles tendon with a normal-appearing ultrasound. The grading includes the following:grade 1—blue (hardest tissue) to green (hard tissue), grade 2—yellow (intermediate tissue), and grade 3—red (soft tissue).[51] In this subset of patients with a symptomatic Achilles tendon, sonoelastography can detect early changes in tissue elasticity related to inflammation. This early inflammation is typically missed by conventional ultrasound. In the paper by Fusini and colleagues,[51] sonoelastography showed a high to excellent sensitivity, specificity, and accuracy in addition to a high degree of agreement with both clinical examination and ultrasound studies.

SUMMARY

Both acute and chronic conditions of the Achilles tendon can be difficult to successfully treat. When looking at outcomes between noninsertional and insertional Achilles tendinopathies the noninsertional pathologies seem to have more successful outcomes. When conservative treatment fails, surgical intervention is the next logical option in the treatment algorithm. With the relative success of conservative treatment with noninsertional Achilles pathology several studies have been focused on the use of biologics in this subset of patients. Because of the spectrum of technologies and difference in techniques as well as the wide variation in biological use, implementation of specific and standardized treatment protocols has not been established.

The combination of advanced Achilles imaging coupled with the activity level and individual patient expectations could assist in the use and potential standardized treatment protocols for patients who have failed conservative treatments.

Biologics in both vitro and vivo studies have shown the ability to upregulate and enhance the natural process of tendon healing. Their use in augmentation in surgical intervention for Achilles tendon pathologies need to continue to be studied and streamlined. Evidence-based treatment protocols and identification of the most effective and appropriate biological treatments of Achilles tendon pathologies will to be determined as more studies and patient outcomes are reported.

CLINICS CARE POINTS

- Orthobiologics in vivo can show an increase in healing potential for Achilles tendon repairs and reconstructions.

- Clinical relevance is still debated as to if and which orthobiologics enhance acute of chronic healing of tendons.
- Further clinical research is necessary.

REFERENCES

1. Sobhani S, Dekker R, Postema K, et al. Epidemiology of ankle and foot overuse injuries in sports: a systematic review. Scand J Med Sci Sports 2013;23:669–86.
2. Khan KM, Cook JL, Bonar F, et al. Histopathology of common tendinopathies. Update and implications for clinical management. Sports Med 1999;27:393–408.
3. Leung JL, Griffith JF. Sonography of chronic Achilles tendinopathy: a case-control study. J Clin Ultrasound 2008;36:27–32.
4. Maffulli N, Longo UG, Maffulli GD, et al. Marked pathological changes proximal and distal to the site of rupture in acute Achilles tendon ruptures. Knee Surg Sports Traumatol Arthrosc 2011;19:680–7.
5. Pingel J, Lu Y, Starborg T, et al. 3-D ultrastructure and collagen compostion of healthy and overloaded human tendon: evidence of tenocyte and matrix buckling. J Anat 2014;224:548–55.
6. Benjamin M, Ralphs JR. Tendons and ligaments-an overview. Histol Histopathol 1997;12:1135–44.
7. Gott M, Ast M, Lane LB, et al. Tendon phenotype shold dicate tissue engineering modality in tendon repair: a review. Discov Med 2011;12:75–84.
8. Docheva D, Muller SA, Majewski M, et al. Bilogics for tendon repair. Adv Drug Deliv Rev 2015;84:222–39.
9. LaPrade RF, Geeslin AG, Murry IR, et al. Biologic treatments for sports injuries II think tank-current concepts. Future research, and barriers to advancement, part 1: biologics overview, ligament injury, tendinopathy. Am J Sports Med 2016;44: 3270–83.
10. Webb WR, Dale TP, Lomas AJ, et al. The application of poly(3-hydroxybutyrate-co-3-hydroxyhexanoate) scaffolds for tendon repair in the rat model. Biomaterials 2013;34:6683–94.
11. Dohan Ehrenfest DM, Rasmusson L, Albrektsson T. Classification of platelet concentrates: from pure platelet-rich plasma (P-PRP) to leucocyte-and platelet-rich fibrin (L-PRF). Trends Biotechnol 2009;27:158–67.
12. Lin MT, Chiang CF, Wu CH, et al. Meta-analysis comparing autologous blood-derived products (including platelet-rich plasma) injection versus placebo in patients with Achilles tendinopathy. Arthroscopy 2018;34:1966–75.
13. Fildardo G, DiMatteo B, Kon E, et al. Platelet-rich plasma in tendon-related disorders: results and indications. Knee Surg Sports Traumatol Arthrosc 2016. https://doi.org/10.1007/s00167-016-4261-4.
14. Imam MA, Holton J, Horriat S, et al. A systemic review of the concept and clinical applications of bone marrow aspirate concentrate in tendon pathology. Sicot J 2017;3:58.
15. Broese M, Toma I, Haasper C, et al. Seeding a human tendon matrix with bone marrow aspirates compared to previously isolated hBMSCs-an in vitro study. Technol Health Care 2011;19:469–79.
16. Sharma P, Maffulli N. Tendon injury and tendinopathy: healing and repair. J Bone Joint Surg Am 2005;87:187–202.

17. Leksa V, Godar S, Shiller HB, et al. TGF-beta-induced apoptosis in endothelial cells mediated by M6P/IGFII-R and mini-plasminogen. J Cell Sci 2005;118: 4577–86.

18. Maeda T, Sakabe T, Sunaga A, et al. Conversion of mechanical force into TGF-beta-mediated biochemical signals. Curr Biol 2011;21:933–41.

19. Jorgensen HG, McLellan SD, Crossan JF, et al. Neutralisation of TGF beta or binding of VLA-4 to fibronectin prevents rat tendon adhesion following transection. Cytokine 2005;30:195–202.

20. Katzet EB, Wolenski M, Loiselle AE, et al. Impact of Smad3 loss of function on scarring and adhesion formation during tendon healing. J Ortho Res 2011;29: 684–93.

21. Potter RM, Huynh RT, Volper BD, et al. Impact of TGF-B inhibition during acute exercise on Achilles tendon extracellular matrix. Am J Physiol Regul Integr Comp Physiol 2017;312:R157–64.

22. Wilgus TA, Ferreira AM, Oberyszyn TM, et al. Regulation of scar formation by vascular endothelial growth factor. Lab Invest 2008;88:579–90.

23. Boyer MI, Watson JT, Lou J, et al. Quantitative variation in vascular endothelial growth factor mRNA expression during early flexor tendon healing: an investigation in a canine model. J Orthop Res 2001;19:869–72.

24. Tempfer H, Kaser-Eichberger A, Lehner C, et al. Bevacizumab improves Achilles tendon repair in rat model. Cell Physiol Biochem 2018;46:1148–58.

25. Wurgler-Hauri CC, Dourte LM, Baradet TC, et al. Temporal expression of 8 growth factors in tendon-to-bone healing in a rat supraspinatus model. J Shoulder Elbow Surg 2007;16:S198–203.

26. Wang XT, Liu PY, Tang JB. Tendon healing in vitro: genetic modification of tenocytes with exogenous PDGF gene and promotion of collagen gene expression. J Hand Surg Am 2004;29:884–90.

27. Thomopoulos S, Zaegel M, Das R, et al. PDGF-BB released in tendon repair using a novel delivery system promotes cell proliferation and collagen remodeling. J Orthop Res 2007;25:1358–68.

28. Thomopoulos S, Das R, Silva MJ, et al. Enhanced flexor tendon healing through controlled delivery of PDGF-BB. J Orthop Res 2009;27:1209–15.

29. Lyras DN, Kazakos K, Georgiadis G, et al. Does a single application of PRP alter the expression of IGF-I in the early phase of tendon healing? J Foot Ankle Surg 2011;50:276–82.

30. Zhang M, Huang B. The multi-differentiation potential of peripheral blood mononuclear cells. Stem Cell Res Ther 2012;3:48.

31. Ogle ME, Segar CE, Sridhar S, et al. Monocytes and macrophages in tissue repair: implications for immunoregenerative biomaterial design. Exp Biol Med (Maywood) 2016;241:1084–97.

32. Forbes SJ, Rosenthal N. Preparing the ground for tissue regeneration: from mechanism to therapy. Nat Med 2014;20:857–69.

33. Kuwana M, Okazaki Y, Kodama H, et al. Human circulating CD14+ monocytes as a source of progenitors that exhibit mesenchymal cell differenciation. J Leukoc Biol 2003;74:833–45.

34. Barnett FH, Rosenfeld M, Wood M, et al. Macrophages form functional vascular mimicry channels in vivo. Sci Rep 2016;6:36659.

35. Barbeck M, Unger RE, Booms P, et al. Monocyte preseeding leads to an increased implant bed vascularization of biphasic calcium phosphate bone substitutes via vessel maturation. J Biomed Mater Res A 2016;104:2928–35.

36. Huk K, Olsen BR. The roles of vascular endothelial growth factor in bone repair and regeneration. Bone 2016;91:30–8.
37. Suckow MA, Hodde JP, Wolter WR, et al. Repair of experimental Achilles tenotomy with porcine renal capsule material in a rat model. J Mater Sci Mater Med 2007;18:1105–10.
38. Ning LJ, Zhang Y, Chen XH, et al. Preparation and characterization of decellularized tendon slices for tendon tissue engineering. J Biomed Mater Res A 2012; 100:1448–56.
39. Farnebo S, Woon CY, Bronstein JA, et al. Decellularized tendon-bone composite grafts for extremity reconstruction: an experimental study. Plast Reconstr Surg 2014;133:79–89.
40. Lohan A, Stoll C, Albrecht M, et al. Human hamstring tenocytes survive when seeded into a decellularized porcine achilees tendon extracellular matrix. Connect Tissue Res 2013;54:305–12.
41. Lee DK. Achilles tendon repair with acellular tissue graft augmentation in neglescted ruptures. J Foot Ankle Surg 2007;46:451–5.
42. Lee DK. A preliminary study on the effects of acellular tissue graft augmentation in acute Achilles tendon ruptures. J Foot Ankle Surg 2008;47:8–12.
43. Wisbeck JM, Parks BG, Schon LC. Xenograft scaffold full-wrap reinformcement of Krackow Achilles tendon repair. Orthopedics 2012;35:e331–4.
44. Gilbert TW, Stewart-Akers AM, Simmons-Byrd A, et al. Degradation and remodeling of small intestinal submucosa in canine Achilles tendon repair. J Bone Joint Surg Am 2007;89:621–30.
45. Zantop T, Gilbert TW, Yoder MC, et al. Extracellular matrix scaffolds are repopulated by bone marrow-derived cells in a mouse model of Achilles tendon reconstruction. J Orthop Res 2006;24:1299–309.
46. Oloff L, Elmi E, Nelson J, et al. Retrospective analysis of the effectiveness of platelet-rich plasma in the treatment of Achilles tendinopathy: pretreatment and posttreatment correlation of magnetic resonance imaging and clinical assessment. Foot Ankle Spec 2015;8:490–7.
47. Albano D, Messina C, Usuelli FG, et al. Magnetic resonance and ultrasound in Achilles tendinopathy: predictive role and response assessment to platelet-rich plasma and adipose-derived stromal vascular fraction injection. Eur J Radiol 2017;95:130–5.
48. Indino C, D'Ambrosi RD, Usuelli FG. Biologics in the treatment of Achilles tendon pathologies. Foot Ankle Clin N Am 2019;24:471–93.
49. Mahoney JM. Imaging techniques and indications. Clin Podiatr Med Surg 2017; 34:115–28.
50. Klauser AS, Miyamoto H, Bellmann-Weiler R, et al. Sonoelastography: musculoskeletal applications. Radiology 2014;272:622–33.
51. Fusini F, Langella F, Busilacchi A, et al. Real-time sonoelastography: principles and clinical applications in tendon disorders. A systematic review. Muscles Ligaments Tendons J 2018;7:467–77.

Biologics in the Treatment of Plantar Fasciitis

Alan Ng, DPM[a,b,]*, Robert Cavaliere, DPM[b], Lauren Molchan, DPM[b]

KEYWORDS

- Biologics • Growth factors • Plantar fasciitis • Regenerative medicine • Stem cells

KEY POINTS

- The role of regenerative medicine in the treatment of musculoskeletal disorders is continually expanding. Biologic therapies are being explored for their regenerative potential in a wide array of musculoskeletal disorders.
- Biologic therapies are categorized based on their derivation into three broad categories: cellular, blood, and noncellular.
- Biologic therapies can provide a multitude of different cellular components, growth factors, and proteins in an attempt to restore normal tissue biology and may be useful as an adjunct in the treatment of recalcitrant plantar fasciitis.

INTRODUCTION

Plantar fasciitis is a one of the most common musculoskeletal (MSK) disorders encountered in a foot and ankle specialist's office, afflicting up to 15% of adults[1] and accounting for up to 1 million patient visits per year.[2] The diagnosis of plantar fasciitis is mostly based on clinical symptoms and specific physical examination findings. Patients usually present with sharp pain isolated to the medial plantar tubercle, plantar calcaneus, or along the medial or central band of the fascia itself. Subjective complaints of post-static dyskinesia and worsening symptoms with barefoot walking are common. Most cases are believed to be secondary to altered biomechanics, which must be addressed. Heel pain of neurologic, arthritic, or traumatic origin should be ruled out as appropriate. Other, more obscure, causes should be explored in chronic cases unresponsive to standard treatment. Most cases of symptomatic plantar fasciitis are resolved with conservative therapies. However, approximately 10% remain recalcitrant.

Plantar fasciitis has historically been considered an acute inflammatory disorder; however, it is now understood that the local histologic findings represent a more

^a Advanced Orthopedic and Sports Medicine Specialists, Denver, CO, USA; ^b Highlands-Presbyterian, St. Luke's Podiatric Medicine and Surgery Residency Program, 1719 East 19th Avenue, Denver, CO 80218, USA
* Corresponding author. Highlands-Presbyterian, St. Luke's Podiatric Medicine and Surgery Residency Program, 1719 East 19th Avenue, Denver, CO 80218.
E-mail address: alan.ng@occ-ortho.com

Clin Podiatr Med Surg 38 (2021) 245–259
https://doi.org/10.1016/j.cpm.2020.12.009
0891-8422/21/© 2020 Elsevier Inc. All rights reserved.

podiatric.theclinics.com

chronic, degenerative state without inflammation.[3] As time progresses, one would expect the normal transition of an acute inflammatory process into one with features of remodeling. From time to time patients may find themselves stuck in a chronic state of cyclical inflammation leading to tissue degeneration, refractory symptoms, and disability. With this understanding, the terms "plantar fasciitis" and "plantar fasciosis" are sometimes used interchangeably. This idea process has influenced the treatment approach of some practitioners who have started to implement the idea of regenerative medicine and use of biologic adjuvants in the treatment of plantar heel pain.

REGENERATIVE MEDICINE AND BIOLOGICS

The term "biologics" refers to a specific class of nonpharmacologic treatments that improve the healing potential of native, damaged tissues. As per the US Food and Drug Administration (FDA), biologic therapies are "sugars, proteins or nucleic acids or complex combinations of these substances, or may be living entities, such as cells and tissues."[4] When discussing the new popularity of regenerative medicine and biologics, it is important to distinguish among blood-derived, cellular-derived, and noncellular therapies. These three categories represent the biologic methods most commonly used in the treatment of orthopedic MSK injuries (**Table 1**).

Cell-derived therapies refer to the introduction of undifferentiated cells directly into local tissues.[5] Blood-derived therapies refer to the local introduction of whole blood or specific blood components to host tissue, providing supraphysiologic concentrations of cytokines and other substances.[6] We define noncellular biologic therapies as the recruitment and influx of growth factors and cytokines in response to mechanical stimulation of local tissues.

This new realm of regenerative medicine focuses on the process of harnessing one's biologic capacity in hopes to restore tissues to their preinjured state (see **Table 1**). The main goals of biologic therapy are as follows:

- Stimulate a healing response
- Modulate further tissue degeneration
- Eliminate pain
- Increase function

CELLULAR THERAPIES
Undifferentiated Cells: What Are They?

An undifferentiated cell has the ability to differentiate and capacity for self-renewal.[7] Self-renewal capacity suggests the ability of cells to proliferate without undergoing biologic aging or loss of its differentiation potential.[8] The ability of a cell to differentiate into different tissue types is dictated by its potency.

Totipotent cells[9] are able to form all cell and tissue types that contribute to the formation of an organism, including extraembryonic and placental cells. By definition,

Table 1 **Biologic therapies**		
Cell Derived	**Blood Derived**	**Noncellular**

Undifferentiated cells from
    Placental tissues
    Bone marrow aspirate
    Adipose tissue
	Platelet-rich plasma	Extracorporeal shockwave

only the embryo itself is classified as such. Pluripotent stem cells have the ability to form any cell type in the body, because they have the ability to expand in vitro and form tissue derived from endoderm, mesoderm, or ectodermal origin.

Only cells that are harvested from the first stages of embryonic development are considered to be pluripotent or totipotent and are referred to as "embryonic" stem cells.[9] Because cells are harvested later on in the stages of embryonic development (10–14 days postfertilization), it is believed that the procured cells are limited to either multipotency or unipotency. Because of this, these cells are commonly referred to as "adult" stem cells.

Multipotent cells[9] are only able to form cells specific to a particular germ layer. There are two main types of multipotent stem cells: hematopoietic and nonhematopoietic cells. Hematopoietic cells are committed to differentiate into cells of blood lineage, whereas nonhematopoietic cells are capable of differentiating into several connective tissue types including osteocytes, adipocytes, chondrocytes, tenocytes, and myoblasts.[10,11] Also known as "mesenchymal" stem cells (MSCs), these nonhematopoietic cells are usually derived from bone marrow, although less commonly they are derived from fat, skin, periosteum, or muscle.[12] MSCs have the advantage of being easily obtainable, and with the appropriate microenvironment, can differentiate into various target tissues.

Sources of Undifferentiated, Multipotent Cells

Placental tissues

The human placenta is a rich source of cells, growth factors, cytokines, and extracellular matrix proteins. It is composed of a variety of different anatomic layers each with their own individual properties, cell types, and proliferative potentials.[13,14] Fetal-derived tissues are well known for their anti-inflammatory, antiscarring, and angiogenic effects and have been shown to exhibit higher proliferative potential than bone marrow–derived cells.[15] These cells are multipotent and have capacity to proliferate into fat, cartilage, bone, skeletal muscle, or neural tissues. They are said to be immunoprivileged, meaning that they can go unrecognized as a foreign body, and serve as a low-risk source of allograft tissue. Up to 1 million cells per gram of tissue can potentially be available for collection.[13]

Amnion-derived tissues can play an important role in the modulation of the inflammatory cascade through multiple mechanisms. They host a variety of different anti-inflammatory proteins, such as interleukin (IL)-1RA and IL-10. These cytokines are responsible for the inhibition of proinflammatory proteins including IL-1, matrix metalloproteinases, and tumor necrosis factor-α. Downregulation of these cytokines have been shown to have a positive effect on macrophages ability to convert from a proinflammatory phenotype to an anti-inflammatory phenotype.[16] High concentrations of hyaluronic acid found throughout amniotic extracellular matrix ECM also contribute to its anti-inflammatory effects.

Anabolic properties of placental-derived cells have been shown in vitro,[17] highlighting their ability to positively influence the deposition of collagen, elastin, and glycosaminoglycans in tenocyte growth mediums. Cells found within amniotic tissues also can promote anticatabolic pathways. This is through increased expression of tissue inhibitors of metalloproteinases. These protease inhibitors serve to inhibit matrix metalloproteinases, limiting the degradation of extracellular matrix protein and ultimately contributing to a regenerative environment ideal for tissue healing.[13]

Harvested placental tissues undergo extensive regulation by the FDA and American Association of Tissue Banks, screening for communicable diseases and ensuring a safe, storable product that is easy to use.[18,19] Once acquired, these tissues undergo enzymatic debridement, separation, decontamination, and preservation. Many different storage techniques are currently available, although dehydrated and cryopreserved allograft products have recently become the preservation methods of choice.[20] These methods, however, are not perfect and may potentially inhibit the tissues biologic composition, cell count, and immunogenicity. Cryopreservation methods have been shown to decrease protein contents within placental tissues, although the effects were minimal and composition was ultimately similar to that of fresh placental tissues.[21] Similarly, dehydration techniques have been shown to have minimal effect on proliferative biologic potential and tensile strength.[22]

Bone marrow aspirate

Bone marrow aspirate (BMA) is easily harvested from the calcaneus, distal or proximal tibia, or iliac crest. BMA contains MSCs and many other cellular components, such as growth factor and ILs that contribute to its regenerative properties. Approximately 0.001% of cells in BMA are MSCs; however, after centrifugation cells may be concentrated six- to seven-fold.[23] BMA concentrate (BMAC) is the term used for this higher concentrated form of MSCs from BMA. BMAC is another source of MSCs that has commonly been used to treat MSK disorders. It has been well documented that multipotent MSCs from BMAC have the capacity to differentiate into a wide range of cell types depending on their surrounding environment and growth factors.

Other cells found within BMAC include a variety of growth factors, such as platelet-derived growth factor, insulin-like growth factor I, granulocyte-macrophage colony–stimulating factor, bone morphogenic proteins 2 and 7, and IL-8 and IL-1 receptor antagonists.[24,25] These markers activate signaling pathways to stimulate cell proliferation, differentiation, and angiogenesis.[23] The signaling cascades generated by these markers ultimately reduce inflammation, fibrosis formation, and apoptosis thereby aiding in the healing process of damaged tissue.

Adipose

There are two types of adipose tissue in the body, brown and white. Brown adipose is primarily found surrounding internal organs and is specialized to retain heat. White adipose is the predominant adipose type in adults and is known to be another rich source of MSCs.[26] These cells were originally described as "preadipocytes" in the 1970s by Dardick and colleagues.[27] Adipose is derived from mesodermal lineage, similar to other tissues of the MSK system. Immature adipose stem cells differentiate into their mature form by a process known as "adipogenesis." This process is ultimately controlled by various signaling pathways generated by the native tissue where the adipose-derived cells are placed. When exposed to a specific tissue type, adipose-derived MSCs have the ability to differentiate into similar cell types of mesenchymal lineage.[26]

Adipose tissue is abundant in MSCs. The highest concentration of MSCs are found within white adipose versus other tissue sources, such as bone marrow, synovium, and skeletal muscle.[28] Isolations of adipose can yield up to 5000 cells per gram of tissue.[29] Because of their high availability in the subcutaneous fat, MSCs are concentrated from the discarded waste of subcutaneous liposuction with minimal donor site morbidity (**Box 1**).

Current Evidence

In 2013, Zelen and colleagues[32] examined the efficacy of micronized dehydrated human amnion/chorion membrane injected as a treatment modality for refractory plantar fasciitis in 45 patients. Results showed a significant improvement in the American Orthopaedic Foot & Ankle Society (AOFAS) scores, in favor of the micronized dehydrated amnion/chorion product versus placebo. These improvements were noticeable within

> **Box 1**
> **Mechanisms of action: undifferentiated, multipotent cells**
>
> - Direct contact with host tissue → cellular engraftment or incorporation and differentiation into native tissue
> - Upregulation of genes when contact injured cells[30]
>   - Anti-inflammation
>   - Transfer vesicles containing mitochondria and microRNA
> - Paracrine effect → signaling between cells to recruit growth factors, cytokines, proteins
>   - IL-1RA, IL-10, tissue inhibitors of metalloproteinases, hyaluronic acid → anti-inflammatory
>   - Angiopoietin-like 4, ANG, acidic fibroblast growth factor → angiogenic
>   - Insulin-like growth factor-binding protein-1, transforming growth factor-b1, insulin-like growth factor-1, hepatocyte growth factor → regenerative
> - Direct secretion of growth factors and cytokines from MSCs[31]
>
> *Data from* Prockop DJ, Oh JY. Mesenchymal stem/stromal cells (MSCs): Role as Guardians of Inflammation. Mol Ther. 2012; 20:14–20; and Caplan AI, Dennis JE. Mesenchymal Stem Cells as Trophic Mediators. J Cell Biochem. 2006; 98:1076–84.

1 week and consistently improved throughout the follow-up period. Similar improvements were found when comparing the patients receiving different volumes of the allograft tissue.

In 2014, Hanselman and colleagues[33] randomized 23 patients and compared the use of a cryopreserved human amniotic membrane with traditional corticosteroid injections to address recalcitrant plantar fasciitis symptoms. Patients had the option to receive one or two injections depending on their perceived course of recovery. No significant differences were found between groups when patients elected to receive a single injection. Patients who elected for a second cryopreserved human amniotic membrane injection relayed greater improvements in pain at 12 weeks compared with the two-injection corticosteroid cohort. These results suggest a dose-dependent effect in regard to foot pain and function.

Werber,[34] in 2015, retrospectively investigated the injection of an amniotic tissue allograft in 44 patients with chronic plantar fasciosis nonresponsive to at least 6 months of traditional conservative care. Patients reported significant improvements in visual analog scale (VAS) scores at 4 weeks, with continued improvements through 12 weeks. At final follow-up, all patients noted that their self-reported pain had reduced from severe to mild.

In 2017, Sun and coworkers[35] reported a case of a 53-year-old woman who had failed conservative and surgical (tendo Achilles lengthening, plantar fasciotomy) therapies to address chronic plantar fasciosis. After 1 year of continued symptoms, the patient underwent revision plantar fasciotomy with application of an intact cryopreserved human placental membrane allograft. After 2 years of continued follow-up, the patient continued to have a satisfactory recovery with a greater than 90% decrease in pain and discomfort.

Cazzell and colleagues,[36] in 2018, conducted a multicenter trial in support of a micronized dehydrated human amnion/chorion membrane injection when compared with a saline placebo in 145 patients. Patients in the treatment group had a 76% reduction in their VAS scores, as compared with a 45% reduction in the placebo group. Of the patients who received the micronized amnion/chorion product, 82.2% reported at least a 50% reduction in their VAS scores from baseline.

The use of BMAC or lipoaspirate-derived therapies in the treatment of plantar fasciitis/fasciosis has yet to be explored. Recent literature primarily focuses on animal studies and other common MSK disorders, highlighting the potential cellular effects as it relates to tissue regeneration and inflammation control. Rat model studies using MSCs from either BMAC or adipose found improved Achilles tendon healing, reduced fibrosis, improved strength, increased organized collagen formation, and improved vascularization.[37–39] Usuelli and colleagues[29] studied adipose-derived MSCs to supplement Achilles repair in human subjects and found tendons supplemented with MSCs had greater improvement in VAS, AOFAS, and VISA-A score compared with platelet-rich plasma (PRP) injected cohort. Similarly, Centeno and colleagues[40] found anterior cruciate ligaments supplemented with BMAC had improved pain and function compared with control subjects. The evidence provided by these in vitro and limited in vivo studies shows promise for MSCs as a viable treatment of plantar fasciitis.

BLOOD-DERIVED THERAPIES
Platelet-Rich Plasma: What Is It?

Platelets are some of the earliest blood-derived cellular elements found at a site of tissue injury and play an extremely important role throughout the stages of wound healing.[6] PRP is defined as a superconcentrated portion of plasma of which the quantity of platelets are greater than baseline levels.[41] This platelet-rich solution is able to contribute to the influx of various growth factors and cytokines, promoting a healing cascade and regenerative effect in injured tissues. To be qualified as platelet rich, plasma levels must have a minimum of five times the normal concentration of platelets. This equates to approximately 1 million platelets per microliters of blood.[42] To date, the exact number of platelets or growth factors required to impart a healing effect is poorly understood. Some studies have suggested the regenerative efficacy of PRP with platelet levels 2.0- to 8.5-fold baseline levels.[43]

To acquire autologous PRP, whole blood is drawn from the cubital vein of the patient. The amount of blood drawn depends on the volume of PRP needed to address particular pathology, although typically 30 to 50 mL of blood is sufficient in the case of a plantar fascia injection. This blood is then introduced into a centrifuging process, separating the blood into three distinct components: (1) plasma layer (platelets), (2) buffy coat layer (white blood cells), and (3) the remaining red blood cell layers. This top-layer plasma coat is then isolated with the use of a syringe and 18-gauge needle, with caution not to disrupt the platelet-poor components of the spun blood.[44,45] The total centrifugal time and number of spin cycles are variable and at the discretion of the provider.[46] After isolation of the PRP, additives, such as calcium citrate or thrombin, are sometimes used to activate the sample, which then stimulates the formation of a clot and the release of growth factors before introduction into a patient. Although some studies show added benefit to thrombin activated platelets versus their inactivated counterpart,[47] there is currently no consensus as to whether or not platelets should be activated and which additive should be used.

The use of PRP in the treatment of plantar fasciitis has been shown to be safe and is routinely performed with minimal complications. In 2016, Chiew and colleagues[46] reviewed 12 relevant articles and found no major complications reported in any of the studies. The most common side effects of PRP therapy seem to be associated with self-limiting local post-treatment pain (**Box 2**).

Current Evidence

In 2014, Mahindra and coworkers[49] sought to compare traditional corticosteroid injections and PRP injections with placebo saline injections in patients with chronic plantar fasciitis symptoms. Patients received 2.5 to 3 mL of single-spun PRP versus equivalent amounts of methylprednisolone or saline injections. There were significantly different improvements in VAS scores and AOFAS scores at 3 weeks and 3 months follow-up in the PRP and corticosteroid groups. There were no improvements in the saline control group at any point in the study period. These results mirror those of the meta-analysis from Yang and colleagues,[50] concluding that there is limited evidence in support of PRP versus corticosteroid injection therapy, despite similar early and intermediate improvement rates.

Monto,[51] in 2014, prospectively followed 40 patients with chronic plantar fasciitis randomized to receive an injection of either DepoMedrol or 3 mL of single-spun PRP. Patients who received the corticosteroid injections experienced early significant improvement in AOFAS scores, although these scores dramatically dropped to baseline at 12 and 24 months follow-up. In contrast, patients receiving the PRP injections not only had significant improvements in AOFAS scores early in follow-up, but these improvements were maintained through the 24-month follow-up period.

Shetty and colleagues,[52] in 2018, conducted a three-arm trial of 90 patients with refractory plantar fasciitis symptoms. Patients were grouped to receive injections of either methylprednisolone acetonide, 2 mL of double-spun PRP, or sterile saline solution. Patients who received the corticosteroid injection showed more significant improvements in pain and limitations scores early in the follow-up (1 month), whereas patients who received the PRP injection showed significantly better improvements in the long term (6, 12, and 18 months). Although patients who received PRP had significantly better improvements at final follow-up, no significant drop off effect was noted in the corticosteroid group. Of note, patients who received the steroid injections were more likely to require a repeat injection and were three times more likely to require open surgical release of the plantar fascia.

In 2016, Vahdatpour and coworkers[53] spoke on the beneficial effects of PRP in patients with chronic plantar fasciitis. Thirty-two patients were randomly assigned to receive either 3 mL of PRP or methylprednisolone. Patients in the PRP group experienced significantly higher pain levels at 1 and 3 months postinjection. These findings were self-limiting, however, because patients who received the PRP reported significantly better function at 6 months when compared with their corticosteroid counterparts. There were no significant differences in fascial thickness based on ultrasonography investigation at any point in the follow-up. These results support the early effects of corticosteroid therapy and delayed beneficial effects of PRP injections to address plantar fasciitis.

Most recently, in 2020, Tabrizi and colleagues[54] evaluated the difference in effects of PRP versus traditional corticosteroid therapy in 32 obese patients with recalcitrant plantar fasciitis. Patients either received an injection of dimethylprednisolone or three separate PRP injections, grouped 3 weeks apart. At 24 weeks follow-up, patients in the corticosteroid group had significantly better pain and functional scores as compared with the patients who received PRP. This study is obviously limited by its short follow-up period, potentially ignoring the delayed benefits associated with PRP.

NONCELLULAR THERAPIES
Extracorporeal Shockwave Therapy: What Is It?

The first use of extracorporeal shockwave therapy (ESWT) for an MSK disorder was in 1993 by Loew and Jurgowski[55] to treat calcific tendonitis in the shoulder. Since then, the uses of ESWT have expanded substantially and it is now routinely used to treat plantar fasciitis. The initial idea behind the use of ESWT for heel pain was to dissolve the heel spur, much like in the treatment of kidney stones.[56] Although this theory has since been disproven, positive patient-reported outcomes have popularized the use of ESWT to address the symptoms of pain and disability associated with plantar fasciitis.

ESWT is a noninvasive treatment using pressure waves directed by a handheld probe through soft tissues to a target site. These waves are focused directly to specific areas of concern in soft tissue or bone. ESWT produces an increase in tissue pressure (from 5–120 MPa) within fractions of a second.[56,57] This is immediately followed by a drop to a negative pressure.[56] This phenomenon is not completely understood; however, there are many proposed hypotheses for the mechanism of action of ESWT. There is evidence available that shows this physical change elicited by ESWT can reduce pain and inflammation and stimulate healing.[58] This indicates tissue can convert mechanical stimulation into biochemical signals. The evidence behind the prevailing theories is summarized in **Box 3**. Future in vivo studies are needed to definitively determine the mechanism of action of ESWT; however, it is likely a combination of these previously reported hypotheses.

Current Evidence

Studies have reported success rates of ESWT for the treatment of plantar fasciitis to range from 48% to 88%.[64,65] Many studies report improved pain and function scores

---

Box 3
Mechanisms of action: ESWT

- Stimulation of C-fibers → release of neuropeptides[59]
  - Vasodilation microcirculation → protein extravasation
  - Stimulation fibroblasts
  - Activation osteoclasts/osteoblasts

- Stimulate release of nitric oxide[60]
  - Analgesic
  - Anti-inflammatory
  - Angiogenic

- Substance P initially increase (6–24 hours) → significantly reduced after 24 hours[61]
  - Lower [Substance P] = decreased pain and inflammation

- Gene expression TGF-b1[62,63]
  - Role in tissue healing

Data from Refs.[59–63]

post-ESWT.[66–68] These effects have been shown to begin at the 2-week mark on average and lasting up to 1 year.[65,69–73]

Many studies have shown no significant difference compared with placebo.[70,74] Some authors have theorized these findings to be secondary to the use of local anesthetic blocks to blind the groups. Local anesthetic has been shown to significantly blunt the trophic effect of ESWT.[59] This could explain why other placebo-based trials did find favorable outcomes in the ESWT treatment arms.[57,75] Thompson and colleagues[76] performed a meta-analysis including six randomized controlled trials and 897 patients and found ESWT to significantly improve heel pain; however, the effect size was small.

Considerations

Patient selection

In regard to biologic therapies, correlations between growth factor concentration, cell counts, and particular patient demographics have been shown. Evanson and colleagues,[77] in 2014, reported that levels of PRP growth factors were significantly higher in subjects younger than 25 years when compared with subjects older than 25. More recently in 2019, Taniguchi and colleagues[78] studied the correlation between patient age, sex, and platelet count on the level of PRP growth factors in 39 healthy volunteers between the ages of 20 and 49. A significant negative correlation between the age of volunteers and concentrations of growth factors was found. Gender failed to show a significant influence. A positive correlation was seen between platelet counts and levels of growth factors. Various studies[79,80] have highlighted drastic changes in total undifferentiated cell counts in older individuals, with a decline from 1/10,000 cells at birth to 1/400,000 cells at age 50. The exact amount of cells required to impart biologic regenerative effects is currently unknown; however, it is theorized that the local tissues response to intervention is likely dose dependent.

With these findings in mind, it is important to recognize that the body's ability to regenerate tissue using autologous cells diminishes over time. It is the author's personal preference that PRP/BMAC/adipose regenerative therapy is used in patients younger than the age of 50. Comorbidities, such as diabetes mellitus, peripheral arterial disease, and obesity, must be considered detrimental to patient outcomes and optimized if possible. Patients with a history of thrombocytopenia or other blood-related disorders should have their platelet counts analyzed to qualify their risk of failed treatment.

Use of Local Anesthetics

Although the combination and direct infiltration of local anesthetics into tissue can provide a great source of lasting pain control for patients, one must proceed with caution in the case of biologics. Many studies highlight the deleterious effects of combining local anesthetics with biologic adjuvants, citing decreased platelet aggregation and antiproliferative effects.[81,82] In addition, the use of local anesthetics has been shown to limit the effectiveness of ESWT.[83] When using biologic therapies, it is the author's personal preference to only anesthetize the skin about the proposed treatment site.

Safety

The use of biologics in the treatment of plantar fasciitis has been shown to be safe and can be routinely performed with minimal complications.[36,46,76] Regardless of modality, the most common side effects seem to be associated with local symptoms of pain, swelling, or bruising, which are self-limiting. Understandably, the harvesting process of autograft biologic sources can potentially lead to donor-site morbidity. Cells acquired from allograft sources should be used in caution in patients with known sensitivity to dimethyl sulfoxide, a common cryopreservative.

FUTURE OF BIOLOGICS IN PLANTAR FASCIITIS

The role of biologics in the treatment of MSK disorders is continually expanding. There are various studies in the works that aim to investigate the true effectiveness, safety, and role of biologic therapy in the treatment of plantar fasciitis. To date, clinicaltrials. org hosts a multitude of relevant studies investigating the use of botulinum toxin, amniotic tissue, photobiomodulation, prolotherapy, PRP and ESWT.

The authors are currently involved in an ongoing multicenter trial comparing the use of a flowable, live cell amnion product with standard of care corticosteroid injection therapy. Results are expected to be published in 2021.

SUMMARY

Orthobiologics encompass a broad category of treatments that focus on the recruitment or stimulation of regenerative tissues to heal MSK pathologies. Most biologics do so through MSCs, growth factor, IL, and cytokine activity or recruitment. There is a role for orthobiologics in the treatment of recalcitrant plantar fasciitis that does not respond to standard conservative care. The evidence behind many of these modalities is ever changing and growing within the literature. Although most therapies have strong in vitro results, the in vivo studies show promise but make no general consensus on recommendations or results. There is no evidence for one biologics' success in resolving plantar heel pain over another at this point in time. Future studies are required to better determine differing biologics outcomes compared with one another. The safety profile of these treatments shows minimal risk with only minor complications. Although these modalities show promise in the treatment of heel pain, cost could be a limiting factor. Although these products are FDA approved, many are not covered by insurance and could cost the patient anywhere from a few hundred dollars to thousands depending on the provider and product used.

CLINICS CARE POINTS

- Although plain film radiographs and ultrasound are the routine imaging modalities of choice to aid in the diagnosis of plantar fasciitis, advanced imaging (MRI, computed tomography) should be considered in recalcitrant cases to rule out any underlying diagnoses, such as an insufficiency fracture, fractured calcaneal spur, subtalar joint pathology, or symptomatic bone marrow edema.

- It is important to understand that the use of biologic therapy should be used as a secondary, adjuvant treatment option and not serve as a primary modality in the treatment of plantar fasciitis. Any biomechanical faults must be addressed before an attempt at biologic therapy.

- Patient selection regarding the use of autologous sources of biologic therapy is crucial. Older patients with many comorbidities exhibit a much lower regenerative capacity than a healthy, younger counterpart. The current authors do not recommend the use of PRP/BMAC/adipose derived stem cells in patients older than 50 years of age.

- Consider avoiding the use of local anesthetic infiltration when using biologics to address plantar fasciitis. Studies have shown decreased regenerative potentials with its coupled use.

- The clinician must be aware of all patients' allergies. Albeit rare, a sensitivity to dimethyl sulfoxide can lead to a multitude of local and systemic side effects.

DISCLOSURE

Dr A. Ng, DPM, FACFAS, is a consultant for Organogenesis.

REFERENCES

1. Rompe JD, Furia J, Weil L, et al. Shock wave therapy for chronic plantar fasciopathy. Br Med Bull 2007;81-82(1):183–208.
2. Riddle DL, Schappert SM. Volume of ambulatory care visits and patterns of care for patients diagnosed with plantar fasciitis: a national study of medical doctors. Foot Ankle Int 2004;25(5):303–10.
3. Lemont H, Ammirati KM, Usen N. Plantar fasciitis: a degenerative process (fasciosis) without inflammation. J Am Podiatr Med Assoc 2003;93(3):234–7.
4. Food and Drug Administration. What are biologics questions and answers. Available at: https://www.fda.gov/about-fda/center-biologics-evaluation-and-research-cber/what-are-biologics-questions-and-answers. Accessed May 12, 2020.
5. Coutu DL, François M, Galipeau J. Mesenchymal stem cells and tissue repair. In: Allan DS, Strunk D, editors. Regenerative therapy using blood-derived stem cells. Humana Press; 2012. p. 35–51.
6. Putman DM, Bell GI, Hess DA. Blood-derived ALDHhi cells in tissue repair. In: Allan DS, Strunk D, editors. Regenerative therapy using blood-derived stem cells. Humana Press; 2012. p. 21–34.
7. Grove JE, Bruscia E, Krause DS. Plasticity of bone marrow-derived stem cells. Stem Cells 2004;22(4):487–500.
8. Morrison SJ, Kimble J. Asymmetric and symmetric stem-cell divisions in development and cancer. Nature 2006;441(7097):1068–74.
9. Menon S, Shailendra S, Renda A, et al. An overview of direct somatic reprogramming: the ins and outs of iPSCs. Iran J Med Sci 2016;17(1):141.
10. Pittenger MF. Multilineage potential of adult human mesenchymal stem cells. Science 1999;284(5411):143–7.
11. Samsonraj RM, Rai B, Sathiyanathan P, et al. Establishing criteria for human mesenchymal stem cell potency: establishing criteria for hMSC potency. Stem Cells 2015;33(6):1878–91.
12. Jacobs SA, Roobrouck VD, Verfaillie CM, et al. Immunological characteristics of human mesenchymal stem cells and multipotent adult progenitor cells. Immunol Cell Biol 2013;91(1):32–9.
13. Hannon C, Yanke A, Farr J. Amniotic tissue modulation of knee pain: a focus on osteoarthritis. J Knee Surg 2019;32(01):026–36.
14. McIntyre JA, Jones IA, Danilkovich A, et al. The placenta: applications in orthopaedic sports medicine. Am J Sports Med 2018;46(1):234–47.
15. Poloni A, Maurizi G, Serrani F, et al. Human AB serum for generation of mesenchymal stem cells from human chorionic villi: comparison with other source and other media including platelet lysate: humanized system to propagate foetal MSCs. Cell Prolif 2012;45(1):66–75.
16. Witherel CE, Yu T, Concannon M, et al. Immunomodulatory effects of human cryopreserved viable amniotic membrane in a pro-inflammatory environment in vitro. Cell Mol Bioeng 2017;10(5):451–62.
17. Kimmerling KA, McQuilling JP, Staples MC, et al. Tenocyte cell density, migration, and extracellular matrix deposition with amniotic suspension allograft: ASA PROMOTES TENDON REPAIR. J Orthop Res 2019;37(2):412–20.

18. Food and Drug Administration. Guidance, compliance & regulatory information: biologics. Available at: https://www.fda.gov/vaccines-blood-biologics/guidance-compliance-regulatory-information-biologics. Accessed May 16, 2020.

19. American Association of Tissue Banks. Regulations for tissue banks. Available at: https://www.aatb.org/regulatory. Accessed May 16, 2020.

20. Riau AK, Beuerman RW, Lim LS, et al. Preservation, sterilization and de-epithelialization of human amniotic membrane for use in ocular surface reconstruction. Biomaterials 2010;31(2):216–25.

21. Tan EK, Cooke M, Mandrycky C, et al. Structural and biological comparison of cryopreserved and fresh amniotic membrane tissues. J Biomater Tissue Eng 2014;4(5):379–88.

22. Koob TJ, Rennert R, Zabek N, et al. Biological properties of dehydrated human amnion/chorion composite graft: implications for chronic wound healing: biological properties of dehydrated human amnion/chorion grafts. Int Wound J 2013; 10(5):493–500.

23. Kim GB, Seo MS, Park WT, et al. Bone marrow aspirate concentrate: its uses in osteoarthritis. Int J Mol Sci 2020;21(9):E3224.

24. Cottom JM, Plemmons BS. Bone marrow aspirate concentrate and its uses in the foot and ankle. Clin Podiatr Med Surg 2018;35(1):19–26.

25. Kim WS, Park BS, Kim HK, et al. Evidence supporting antioxidant action of adipose-derived stem cells: protection of human dermal fibroblasts from oxidative stress. J Dermatol Sci 2008;49:133–42.

26. Minteer D, Marra KG, Rubin JP. Adipose-derived mesenchymal stem cells: biology and potential applications. Adv Biochem Eng Biotechnol 2013;129: 59–71.

27. Dardick I, Poznanski WJ, Waheed I, et al. Ultrastructural observations on differentiating human preadipocytes cultured in vitro. Tissue Cell 1976;8(3):561–71.

28. Lee HC, An SG, Lee HW, et al. Safety and effect of adipose tissue-derived stem cell implantation in patients with critical limb ischemia: a pilot study. Circ J 2012; 76:1750–60.

29. Usuelli FG, D'Ambrosi R, Maccario C, et al. Adipose-derived stem cells in orthopaedic pathologies. Br Med Bull 2017;124(1):31–5.

30. Prockop DJ, Oh JY. Mesenchymal stem/stromal cells (MSCs): role as guardians of inflammation. Mol Ther 2012;20:14–20.

31. Caplan AI, Dennis JE. Mesenchymal stem cells as trophic mediators. J Cell Biochem 2006;98:1076–84.

32. Zelen CM, Poka A, Andrews J. Prospective, randomized, blinded, comparative study of injectable micronized dehydrated amniotic/chorionic membrane allograft for plantar fasciitis: a feasibility study. Foot Ankle Int 2013;34(10):1332–9.

33. Hanselman AE, Tidwell JE, Santrock RD. Cryopreserved human amniotic membrane injection for plantar fasciitis: a randomized, controlled, double-blind pilot study. Foot Ankle Int 2015;36(2):151–8.

34. Werber B. Amniotic tissues for the treatment of chronic plantar fasciosis and Achilles tendinosis. J Sports Med 2015;2015:1–6.

35. Sun XP, Wilson AG, Michael GM. Open surgical implantation of a viable intact cryopreserved human placental membrane for the treatment of recalcitrant plantar fasciitis: case report with greater than 2-year follow-up duration. J Foot Ankle Surg 2018;57(3):583–6.

36. Cazzell S, Stewart J, Agnew PS, et al. Randomized controlled trial of micronized dehydrated human amnion/chorion membrane (dHACM) injection compared to placebo for the treatment of plantar fasciitis. Foot Ankle Int 2018;39(10):1151–61.

37. Urdzikova LM, Sedlacek R, Suchy T, et al. Human multipotent mesenchymal stem cells improve healing after collagenase tendon injury in the rat. Biomed Eng Online 2014;13:42.

38. Adams SB Jr, Thorpe MA, Parks BG, et al. Stem cell-bearing suture improves Achilles tendon healing in a rat model. Foot Ankle Int 2014;35(3):292–9.

39. Kenaya A, Deie M, Adachi N, et al. Intra-articular injection of mesenchymal stromal cells in partially torn anterior cruciate ligaments in a rat model. Arthroscopy 2007;35:962–79.

40. Centeno C, Pitts J, Al-Sayegh H, et al. Efficacy of autologous bone marrow concentrate for knee osteoarthritis with and without adipose graft. Biomed Res Int 2014;2014:370621.

41. Marx RE. Platelet-rich plasma (PRP): what is PRP and what is not PRP? Implant Dent 2001;10(4):225–8.

42. Ra Hara G, Basu T. Platelet-rich plasma in regenerative medicine. Biomedical Research and Therapy 2014;1(1):25–31.

43. Smith SE, Roukis TS. Bone and wound healing augmentation with platelet-rich plasma. Clin Podiatr Med Surg 2009;26(4):559–88.

44. Soomekh DJ. Current concepts for the use of platelet-rich plasma in the foot and ankle. Clin Podiatr Med Surg 2011;28(1):155–70.

45. Scioli MW. Platelet-rich plasma injection for proximal plantar fasciitis. Tech Foot Ankle Surg 2011;10(1):7–10.

46. Chiew S, Ramasamy T, Amini F. Effectiveness and relevant factors of platelet-rich plasma treatment in managing plantar fasciitis: a systematic review. J Res Med Sci 2016;21(1):38.

47. Scherer SS, Tobalem M, Vigato E, et al. Nonactivated versus thrombin-activated platelets on wound healing and fibroblast-to-myofibroblast differentiation in vivo and in vitro. Plast Reconstr Surg 2012;129(1):46e–54e.

48. Souza D. Platelet-rich plasma. In: Peng P, Finlayson R, Lee SH, et al, editors. Ultrasound for interventional pain management. Springer International Publishing; 2020. p. 317–24.

49. Mahindra P, Yamin M, Selhi HS, et al. Chronic plantar fasciitis: effect of platelet-rich plasma, corticosteroid, and placebo. Orthopedics 2016;39(2):e285–9.

50. Yang W, Han Y, Cao X, et al. Platelet-rich plasma as a treatment for plantar fasciitis: a meta-analysis of randomized controlled trials. Medicine 2017;96(44): e8475.

51. Monto RR. Platelet-rich plasma efficacy versus corticosteroid injection treatment for chronic severe plantar fasciitis. Foot Ankle Int 2014;35(4):313–8.

52. Shetty SH, Dhond A, Arora M, et al. Platelet-rich plasma has better long-term results than corticosteroids or placebo for chronic plantar fasciitis: randomized control trial. J Foot Ankle Surg 2019;58(1):42–6.

53. Vahdatpour B, Kianimehr L, Ahrar M. Autologous platelet-rich plasma compared with whole blood for the treatment of chronic plantar fasciitis; a comparative clinical trial. Adv Biomed Res 2016;5(1):84.

54. Tabrizi A, Dindarian S, Mohammadi S. The effect of corticosteroid local injection versus platelet-rich plasma for the treatment of plantar fasciitis in obese patients: a single-blind, randomized clinical trial. J Foot Ankle Surg 2020;59(1):64–8.

55. Loew M, Jurgowski W. Initial experiences with extracorporeal shockwave lithotripsy (ESWL) in treatment of tendinosis calcarea of the shoulder. Z Orthop Ihre Grenzgeb 1993;131(5):470–3.

56. Yalcin E, Keskin Akca A, Selcuk B, et al. Effects of extracorporeal shock wave therapy on symptomatic heel spurs: a correlation between clinical outcome and radiologic changes. Rheumatol Int 2012;32(2):343–7.

57. Rompe JD, Hopf C, Nafe B, et al. Low-energy extracorporeal shock wave therapy for painful heel: a prospective controlled single-blind study. Arch Orthop Trauma Surg 1996;115:75–9.

58. Notarnicola A, Moretti B. The biological effects of extracorporeal shock wave therapy (ESWT) on tendon tissue. Muscles Ligaments Tendons J 2012;2(1):33–7.

59. Klonschinski T, Ament SJ, Schlereth T, et al. Application of local anesthesia inhibits effects of low-energy extracorporeal shock wave treatment (ESWT) on nociceptors. Pain Med 2011;12(10):1532–7.

60. Loew M, Rompe JD. Stosswellenbehandlung bei orthopädischen Erkrankungen. Stuttgart (Germany): Enke Verlag; 1998. p. 8–9.

61. Hausdorf J, Schmitz C, Averbeck B, et al. Molecular basis for pain mediating properties of extracorporeal shock waves. Schmerz 2004;18(6):492–7.

62. Banes AJ, Horesovsky G, Larson C, et al. Mechanical load stimulates expression of novel genes in vivo and in vitro in avian flexor tendon cells. Osteoarthr Cartil 1999;7:141–53.

63. Caminoto EH, Alves AL, Amorim RL, et al. Ultrastructural and immunocytochemical evaluation of the effects of extracorporeal shock wave treatment in the hind limbs of horses with experimentally induced suspensory ligament desmitis. Am J Vet Res 2005;66(5):892–6.

64. Ogden JA, Alvarez RG, Marlow M. Shockwave therapy for chronic proximal plantar fasciitis: a meta-analysis. Foot Ankle Int 2002;23:301–8.

65. Rompe JD, Küllmer K, Vogel J, et al. Extracorporeal shock-wave therapy: experimental basis, clinical application. Orthopade 1997;26:215–28.

66. Ragab EM, Othman AM. Platelets rich plasma for treatment of chronic plantar fasciitis. Arch Orthop Trauma Surg 2012;132:1065–70.

67. Gerdesmeyer L, Frey C, Vester J, et al. Radial extracorporeal shock wave therapy is safe and effective in the treatment of chronic recalcitrant plantar fasciitis: results of a confirmatory randomized placebo controlled multicenter study. Am J Sports Med 2008;36:2100–9.

68. Speed CA, Nichols D, Wies J, et al. Extracorporeal shock wave therapy for plantar fasciitis: a double blind randomised controlled trial. J Orthop Res 2003; 21:937–40.

69. Rompe JD. Repetitive low-energy shock wave treatment is effective for chronic symptomatic plantar fasciitis. Knee Surg Sports Traumatol Arthrosc 2007;15:107.

70. Speed CA. Extracorporeal shock-wave therapy in the management of chronic soft-tissue conditions. J Bone Joint Surg Br 2004;86:165–71.

71. Vulpiani MC, Trischitta D, Trovato P, et al. Extracorporeal shock wave therapy (ESWT) in Achilles tendinopathy. A long-term follow-up observational study. J Sports Med Phys Fitness 2009;49:171–6.

72. Saxena A, Fournier M, Gerdesmeyer L, et al. Comparison between extracorporeal shockwave therapy, placebo ESWT and endoscopic plantar fasciotomy for the treatment of chronic plantar heel pain in the athlete. Muscles Ligaments Tendons J 2013;2:312–6.

73. Ugurlar M, Sonmez MM, Ugurlar PY, et al. Effectiveness of four different treatment modalities in the treatment of chronic plantar fasciitis during a 36-month follow-up period: a randomized controlled trial. J Foot Ankle Surg 2018;57(5):913–8.

74. Buchbinder R, Ptasznik R, Gordon J, et al. Ultrasound guided extracorporeal shock wave therapy for plantar fasciitis: a randomized controlled trial. JAMA 2002;288:1364–72.

75. Haake M, Buch M, Schoellner C, et al. Extracorporeal shock wave therapy for plantar fasciitis: randomised controlled multicentre trial. BMJ 2003;327:75–9.

76. Thompson CE, Crawford F, Murray GD. The effectiveness of extra corporeal shock wave therapy for plantar heel pain: a systematic review and meta-analysis. BMC Musculoskelet Disord 2005;6:19.

77. Evanson JR, Guyton MK, Oliver DL, et al. Gender and age differences in growth factor concentrations from platelet-rich plasma in adults. Mil Med 2014;179(7): 799–805.

78. Taniguchi Y, Yoshioka T, Sugaya H, et al. Growth factor levels in leukocyte-poor platelet-rich plasma and correlations with donor age, gender, and platelets in the Japanese population. J Exp Orthop 2019;6(1):4.

79. Melick G, Hayman N, Landsman AS. Mesenchymal stem cell applications for joints in the foot and ankle. Clin Podiatr Med Surg 2018;35(3):323–30.

80. Schipper BM, Marra KG, Zhang W, et al. Regional anatomic and age effects on cell function of human adipose-derived stem cells. Ann Plast Surg 2008;60(5): 538–44.

81. Bausset O, Magalon J, Giraudo L, et al. Impact of local anaesthetics and needle calibres used for painless PRP injections on platelet functionality. Muscles Ligaments Tendons J 2014;4(1):18–23.

82. Lucchinetti E, Awad AE, Rahman M, et al. Antiproliferative effects of local anesthetics on mesenchymal stem cells: potential implications for tumor spreading and wound healing. Anesthesiology 2012;116(4):841–56.

83. Labek G, Auersperg V, Ziernhold M, et al. Influence of local anesthesia and energy level on the clinical outcome of extracorporeal shock wave treatment of chronic plantar fasciitis. Z Orthop Ihre Grenzgeb 2005;143:240–6.

Neglected Achilles Tendon Ruptures

James M. Cottom, DPM, FACFAS*, Charles A. Sisovsky, DPM, AACFAS

KEYWORDS

- Primary achilles repair • V-Y advancement • Turndown flap • FHL tendon transfer
- FDL tendon transfer • Peroneus brevis tendon transfer • Allograft

KEY POINTS

- There are multiple techniques to treat tendon defects in the event that end-to-end repair cannot be achieved after débridement. In general, the choice of treatment technique is based on the size of the resultant gap and the surgeon's comfort with each technique.
- Patients should be counseled on the likelihood of generalized calf atrophy and ankle plantarflexion strength deficits compared with the uninjured side.
- Patients typically return to preinjury status and can perform leisure and sports activities without issues.

Video content accompanies this article at http://www.podiatric.theclinics.com/.

INTRODUCTION

Achilles tendon pathology is a common ailment affecting a wide variety of the population.[1] Early diagnosis and prompt treatment of an acute injury generally result in a more favorable outcome. That said, as common as these injuries are, 25% of ruptures are missed during initial examination.[2] Of these that are missed, most patients present with long-standing pain with the inability to perform normal activities without difficulty. Not all neglected Achilles tendon injuries, however, require surgery. Those who are unable to undergo surgery due to comorbidities or those who have sedentary lifestyles can be treated with custom ankle-foot orthoses.

There are many different surgical techniques and strategies used for Achilles tendon ruptures. The Kuwada[3] classification for Achilles tendon ruptures is one of the most widely used and is useful in deciding which strategy to use based on the size of the deficit (**Table 1**). In this classification, type I lesions are described as partial ruptures less than 50%. These typically are treated conservatively. Type II lesions are complete

Florida Orthopedic Foot and Ankle Center, 1630 South Tuttle Avenue, Sarasota, FL 34239, USA
* Corresponding author.
E-mail address: jamescottom300@hotmail.com

Clin Podiatr Med Surg 38 (2021) 261–277
https://doi.org/10.1016/j.cpm.2020.12.010
0891-8422/21/© 2021 Elsevier Inc. All rights reserved.

Table 1	
Kuwada classification for Achilles tendon ruptures	
Defect Size	**Surgical Procedure**
Partial, 50% tear	Immobilization
≤3 cm	End-to-end anastomosis
3–6 cm	V-Y lengthening ± tendon transfer
>6 cm	Tendon transfer with V-Y advancement or turndown flap

ruptures with a gap measuring less than or equal to 3 cm. Defects of this size are treated with end-to-end anastomosis. Type III lesions are complete ruptures with a tendinous gap measuring between 3 cm and 6 cm. These injuries typically require a tendon/synthetic graft. Lastly, type IV lesions are complete ruptures with a tendinous gap measuring greater than 6 cm. These injuries often require tendon graft with possible V-Y advancement or gastrocnemius recession.[3]

PRIMARY REPAIR

For those injuries less than 3 cm, a primary, end-to-end anastomosis is recommended. Currently, there are only a few techniques in the literature for this type of repair: open, mini-open, or percutaneous. Percutaneous repair is gaining popularity because this reduces the chances of wound dehiscence and infection. With advances in biologics, however, open repairs are healing with fewer complications.[4]

To perform a primary repair, the patient is positioned in the prone position with the feet elevated on pillows. Both extremities are prepped in order to compare the strength and tension of the repair to the contralateral extremity. For primary repairs, the authors recommend the percutaneous technique. A vertical incision is made directly over the ruptured tendon. It is important to débride the ruptured ends of the Achilles tendon because they have been shown to have marked collagen degeneration and disordered arrangement of collagen fibers.[5] Once adequate débridement has occurred, the tendon is grasped with an Allis clamp. The inner arms of the percutaneous system are placed deep to the paratenon on either side of the Achilles tendon. Next, the proximal stump of the Achilles is sutured per manufacturer protocol.

Attention then is directed distally, where a 1-cm incision is made medially and laterally and the posterosuperior aspect of the calcaneus is identified. A hemostat is used to dissect down to the periosteum. A periosteal incision is made at the calcaneus for preparation of anchoring the suture ends into the calcaneus. Next, a nitinol suture passer is passed from the distal incisions, through the distal stump of the Achilles, exiting the midportion of the distal stump. All suture ends from the proximal stump are gathered and passed through the distal tendon stump. The ankle then is placed in an appropriate amount of plantarflexion and the ends of the sutures are anchored within the calcaneus. The paratenon is closed in order to prevent adhesions and the skin is closed in layers using absorbable and nonabsorbable sutures. When using this technique, if after débridement of the tendon rupture there is a gap between 3 cm and 6 cm, the authors likely would perform a flexor hallucis longus (FHL) transfer. If that is the case, the incision needs to be extended as deemed necessary. This technique is described later.

In the technique, described previously, Hsu and colleagues[6] compared the Percutaneous Achilles Repair System (PARS) (Arthrex, Naples, FL) to open repair and found a significant reduction in total complications (5% vs 10.6%, respectively), with improved rates of return to baseline activity. Similarly, McWilliam and Mackay[7] presented their early outcomes utilizing the *Internal*Brace (Arthrex) and reported that the Achilles Tendon Total Rupture Score was 94 ± 14, calf circumference difference was 0.8 cm ± 0.5 cm, and the average time for return to previous/desired level of activity was 18.2 weeks (range 9–26 weeks). They also reported no wound complications, nerve injuries, or reruptures.

Cottom and colleagues[8] presented a biomechanical study in 2017, comparing Krackow repair, traditional PARS repair, and modified PARS repair with additional suture anchors placed into the calcaneus. The specimens were placed through 10 cycles, 500 cycles, and 1000 cycles using the 8871 device (Instron, High Wycombe, United Kingdom). Their results showed a statistically significant difference between all groups after 1000 cycles (P = .040). They concluded that the modified PARS repair using suture anchors placed into the calcaneus proved to be stronger and, possibly, a more reliable construct that might translate to a faster return to activity and be more resistant to an early and aggressive rehabilitation protocol.[8]

V-Y TENDON ADVANCEMENT

The V-Y tendinous flap was first described by Abraham and Pankovich,[9] in 1975, to achieve end-to-end anastomosis of the tendon ends in neglected ruptures. An inverted V-shaped incision is made at the proximal part of the Achilles tendon near the musculotendinous junction. Each arm of the V should measure at least 1.5-times to 2-times the size of the gap, with a larger arm for larger defects.[10] The distal portion of the cut tendon then is advanced until the proximal and distal tendon stump are approximated, without separating the tendon from the underlying muscle. Repair of the tendon stumps is performed using Krackow sutures and no. 5 nonabsorbable polyfilament suture, followed by repair of the proximal tendon in a Y-shaped fashion with 0# braided suture.

In the study by Elias and colleagues,[10] they reported on 15 consecutive patients who underwent V-Y lengthening in conjunction with an FHL tendon transfer for tendon gaps of 5 cm or larger. They found American Orthopaedic Foot and Ankle Society scores were all good to excellent, with an average score of 94.1 of 100. All patients were satisfied with their outcomes (rated good or very good).

TURNDOWN FLAP

The turndown flap was first introduced by Christensen, in 1953,[11] which is used for moderate-sized defects as well as for reinforcement of primary repairs. Since its inception, other variations also have been described, either performed independently or in conjunction with other techniques.[12–14]

A posterior longitudinal incision is made centered over the Achilles tendon. The tendon defect is exposed through sharp dissection of the paratenon. If a turndown flap is deemed necessary after inspection of the tendon gap, the length of the flap is determined by measuring the size of the defect. Although there is no standardized technique for determining the exact graft length, Sanada and Uchiyama[15] suggest preoperatively assessing the contralateral unaffected lower extremity to determine resting gravity ankle plantarflexion with the knee flexed at 90°. By performing the same maneuver on the injured extremity, the true gap distance and, thus, length of flap harvest then can be determined.[15]

TENDON TRANSFERS
Flexor Hallucis Longus

Multiple tendon transfers have been described for the treatment of chronic Achilles tendon ruptures. In 1993, Wapner and colleagues[16] described transferring the FHL tendon through a medial midfoot incision to the calcaneus, anterior to the Achilles insertion with satisfactory results. The FHL tendon is the most commonly used donor for tendon transfer due to its biomechanical strength, phase of action, and line of pull.[17]

To perform this technique, it is the authors' preferred technique to start with placing the patient in a prone position with a well-padded ipsilateral thigh tourniquet inflated to 300 mm Hg. A 10-cm direct posterior or posteromedial longitudinal incision is made over the Achilles tendon to the calcaneal insertion and is taken full thickness down to the level of the paratenon (**Fig. 1**). Care is taken to retract the sural nerve if encountered. The paratenon is incised longitudinally, off-center from the skin incision to prevent adhesions. The paratenon is tagged with Vicryl suture for later repair. At this point, sharp débridement is performed of any diseased tendon until only healthy tissue remains. If the gap is between 3 cm and 6 cm, the decision is made for FHL tendon transfer (**Fig. 2**). It is the authors' preferred technique to utilize a single-incision approach. The deep posterior compartment is incised, exposing the FHL muscle belly, which is confirmed with dorsiflexion and plantarflexion of the hallux. After proper identification, the muscle is followed distally until the tendon is fully formed. The posterior tibial artery and nerve are identified and carefully retracted medially. While plantarflexing the hallux, the FHL tendon is cut as far distal as possible from the single posterior incision. The tendon stump is then whip-stitched utilizing #0 FiberLoop suture (Arthrex) (**Fig. 3**). The suture loop is cut and the ends are passed through the Mini DX Cortical Button (Arthrex).

A guide wire for the Mini DX Cortical Button then is driven from the superior aspect of the calcaneus, bicortically, aiming 1-cm distal to the weight-bearing surface of the

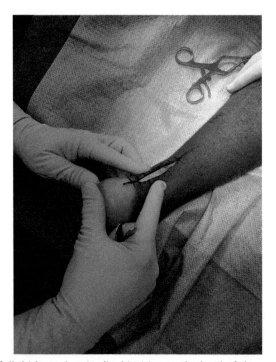

Fig. 1. A 10-cm, full-thickness longitudinal incision to the level of the paratenon.

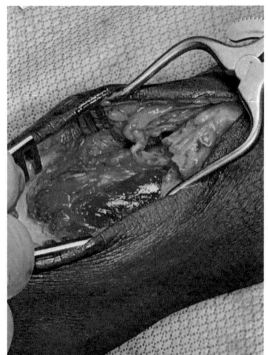

Fig. 2. Tendon gap of 6 cm warranting FHL tendon transfer.

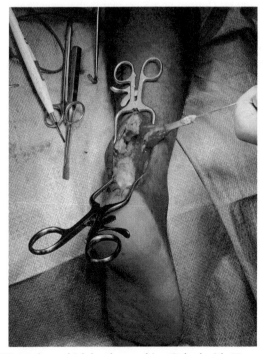

Fig. 3. Harvested FHL tendon, which has been whip-stitched with #0 nonabsorbable suture.

plantar heel (**Fig. 4**). The ideal location for the wire is just distal to the attachment of the plantar fascia at the medial tuber and centrally located within the body of the calcaneus. Care is taken to not drive the guide wire through the plantar fascia or plantar skin. Next, a tendon sizer is utilized to identify the correct size of the biotenodesis screw that will be inserted (**Fig. 5**). The corresponding reamer is then inserted over the guide wire and the calcaneus is reamed, with care taken to leave the plantar cortex intact (**Fig. 6**). The guide wire is removed and the Mini DX Cortical Button is passed through the bone tunnel. After the Mini DX Cortical Button has passed the plantar calcaneal cortex, the button passer is engaged, flipping the button and the passer is removed (**Fig. 7**). Utilizing the tension slide technique, the ends of the FiberLoop suture are pulled, passing the FHL tendon through the bone tunnel until adequate tension has been achieved while positioning the foot in 10° of plantarflexion (Video 1). Next, 1 arm of the FiberLoop suture stitched through the FHL tendon and tied to the other suture. This essentially secures the cortical button on the plantar aspect of the calcaneus. Next, the corresponding biotenodesis screw with a suture passer and the screw is inserted, while keeping tension on the suture ends (**Fig. 8**). Attention then is directed distally, where a nitinol suture passer is passed from the through the distal stump of the Achilles exiting the midportion of the distal stump (**Fig. 9**). All suture ends from the proximal stump are gathered and passed through the distal tendon stump (**Fig. 10**). The ankle then is placed in an appropriate amount of plantarflexion and the ends of the sutures are anchored within the calcaneus (**Fig. 11**). The FHL muscle belly then is sutured into the deep surface of the Achilles tendon (**Fig. 12**). It is optional to use allograft to wrap around the tendon to augment the repair (**Fig. 13**). Finally, the paratenon is reapproximated and the wound is closed in a layered fashion. The patient then is immobilized in a non–weight-bearing splint placed into a slight gravity equinus. This technique was described and adopted from Shinabarger and colleagues.[18]

In a cadaveric study by Cottom and Sisovsky,[19] the investigators found that Ultimate Load proved more favorable in the interference screw with the Mini DX Button group. In their study, they compared 10 matched cadaver specimens. Samples were prepared using 20–pounds per cubic foot (PCF) foam block with a 3-mm thick 40-PCF laminate layer (Sawbones Pacific Research, Vashon Island, Washington). Bovine tendons (Advanced Tissue Concepts, Smithfield, Utah) were trimmed to 6.5-mm diameter and whip-stitched with #2 suture (FiberLoop) (see **Fig. 9**). Mechanical

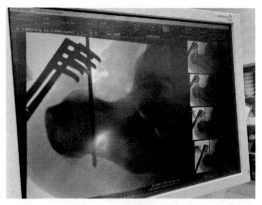

Fig. 4. Guidewire for suture button, which should be 1 cm distal to tuberosity of the calcaneus.

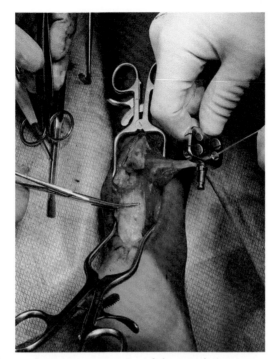

Fig. 5. Tendon sizer to determine correct size of the tenodesis screw.

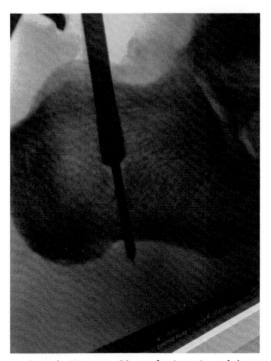

Fig. 6. Reaming approximately 15 mm to 20 mm for insertion of the tenodesis screw.

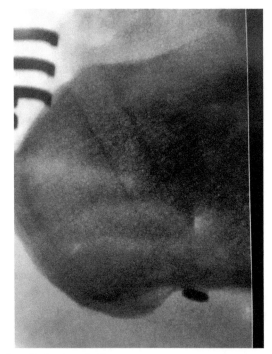

Fig. 7. Insertion of cortical suture button.

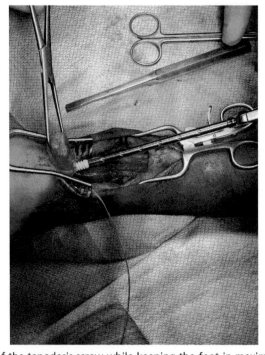

Fig. 8. Insertion of the tenodesis screw while keeping the foot in maximal plantarflexion.

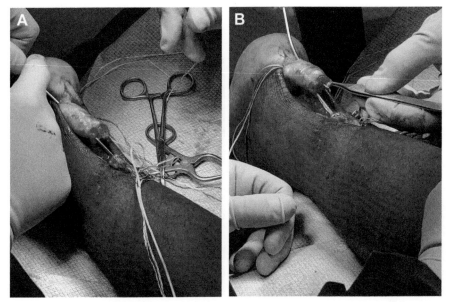

Fig. 9. Nitinol suture passer passing (*A*) through distal-lateral stump and (*B*) through the distal-medial stump in order to gather sutures proximally.

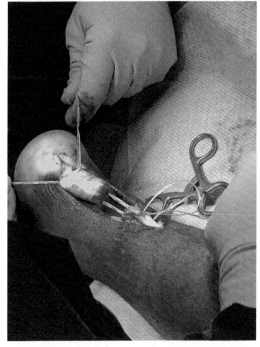

Fig. 10. All suture ends gathered distally in order for proper reapproximation of the tendon ends.

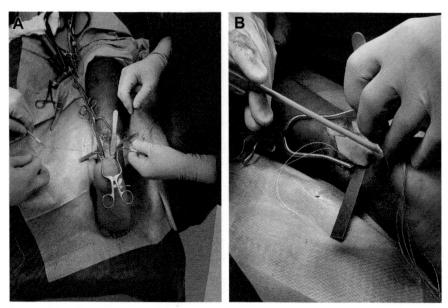

Fig. 11. (*A*) Utilizing Adson pickups to maintain visualization of the anchor locations. (*B*) Insertion of anchors. This is the modified percutaneous technique anchoring the sutures into the calcaneus.

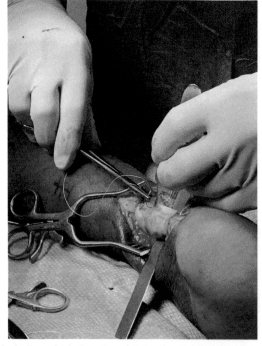

Fig. 12. FHL muscle belly, which is sutured into the Achilles tendon once the repair is complete.

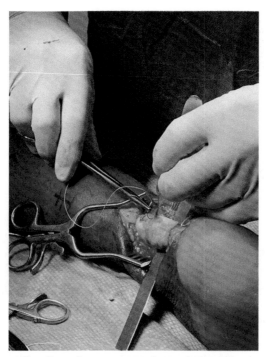

Fig. 13. Optional use of a allograft to augment the tendon repair.

testing was performed using an 8871 Servohydraulic Testing Machine with a 5-kN load cell (Instron, Norwood, Massachusetts) (**Fig. 14**). A vise clamp was used to hold the free end of the tendon to the actuator and the foam block was held to the testing surface using a metal box fixture (**Fig. 15**). Samples loaded were between 20N and 60N for 100 cycles at 1 Hz. Cyclic loading was followed by a pull to failure conducted at 1.25 mm/s. Load and displacement data were recorded at 500 Hz. The mode of failure was recorded at the time of testing. Student *t* tests were used to compare the ultimate load and cyclic displacement results for the 2 repair groups (**Tables 2** and **3**); 90% (n = 9) of failures in group 1 occurred by the suture tearing through the tendon and 10% by the tendon and suture slipping past the screw. Comparatively, 50% (n = 5) of failure in group 2 occurred by the suture tearing through the tendon and the other 50% by the tendon and sutures slipping past the screw. The investigators found that the interference and cortical button both act as fail-safes so if one were to fail, the other acted as a back-up. Knowing this may give surgeons the confidence to allow their patients to bear weight earlier, which ultimately translates into earlier functional rehabilitation. The investigators conclude that this novel technique is one of the more advanced ways to repair neglected Achilles tendon ruptures. Ultimately, there is less bulk at the repair site compared with a turndown flap, the FHL muscle belly provides increased vascular supply to an already hypovascular tendon, and this technique negates the chance of donor site morbidity because harvesting an autograft (ie, hamstring autograft) is not necessary.

Flexor Digitorum Longus

Flexor digitorum longus tendon transfers can be used as an alternative to FHL tendon transfers. To perform this technique, as described by de Cesar Netto and

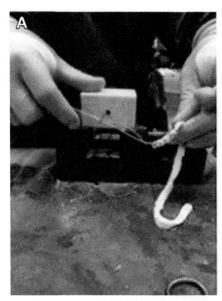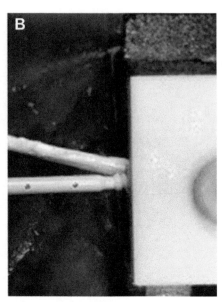

Fig. 14. (*A*) Trimmed tendons whip-stitched with #2 nonabsorbable suture. (*B*) Tenodesis screw inserted, which acts as a fail-safe mechanism.

colleagues,[19] Patients are placed in a semilateral position, with the operative side down, allowing access to both the posterior and medial aspects of the foot and ankle. Those patients who have had prior surgery on the same Achilles tendon through a posterior midline approach are placed in the prone position. Exposure of the Achilles tendon is performed via a posteromedial incision, except in patients who have had prior midline posterior approach. Dissection is performed down to the paratenon with minimal undermining to preserve a full-thickness flap for closure. After proper exposure and opening of the paratenon, tendinopathic tissue is identified and fibrotic and diseased areas of the tendon are resected and/or débrided. A 2-cm to 3-cm separate incision is made longitudinally over the medial aspect of the foot just over the sustentaculum tali, inferiorly to the talar neck. After proper identification of the tibialis posterior tendon sheath, dissection is carried out deep and inferior to it aiming to isolate the FDL tendon. A clamp then is passed underneath the FDL tendon and the

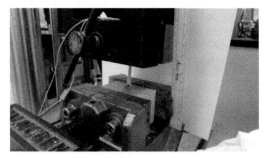

Fig. 15. Vise clamp was used to hold the free end of the tendon to the actuator and the foam block was held to the testing surface.

Table 2
Results of Mini DX Cortical Button plus biotenodesis screw

				Group 1 with Mini DX Cortical Button	
Sample	Ultimate Load (Newtons [N])	Yield Load (N)	Stiffness (N/mm)	Cyclic Displacement (mm)	Mode of failure
1	399	235	98	0.9	Suture tore through tendon
2	464	464	83	0.6	Suture tore through tendon
3	520	234	96	1.1	Suture tore through tendon
4	366	179	84	0.9	Suture tore through tendon
5	350	332	65	1.5	Suture tore through tendon
6	312	237	54	1.6	Suture tore through tendon
7	482	379	69	1.5	Tendon and sutures slipped past screw
8	356	351	67	1.5	Suture tore through tendon
9	409	409	71	3.7	Suture tore through tendon
10	397	217	82	1.2	Suture tore through tendon
Average	406	304	77	1.5	
SD	65	96	14	0.9	

lesser toes are moved to confirm that the appropriate tendon is identified. An additional proximal medial incision is made 6 cm to 10 cm above the tip of medial malleolus at the posterior border of the tibia. After the sheath of the posterior compartment of the leg is opened, the FDL tendon is identified by moving the lesser toes. The FDL tendon then is transected under direct visualization at the distal incision, with the toes in maximum plantar flexion, proximally to the knot of Henry. The FDL tendon stump is delivered carefully through the proximal medial incision, leaving its muscle belly intact. A clamp is used to create a subcutaneous tunnel connecting the proximal medial and

Table 3
Results of solitary biotenodesis screw

				Group 2 with solitary biotenodesis screw	
Sample	Ultimate Load (N)	Yield Load (N)	Stiffness (N/mm)	Cyclic Displacement (mm)	Mode of Failure
1	327	327	86	1.3	Suture tore through tendon
2	347	256	92	1.0	Suture tore through tendon
3	284	204	77	1.7	Suture tore through tendon
4	488	354	81	1.1	Tendon and sutures slipped past screw
5	350	293	93	0.8	Tendon and sutures slipped past screw
6	268	200	84	1.3	Tendon and sutures slipped past screw
7	347	280	75	1.3	Suture tore through tendon
8	432	300	85	1.1	Tendon and sutures slipped past screw
9	380	380	81	1.6	Suture tore through tendon
10	174	241	73	1.4	Tendon and sutures slipped past screw
Average	340	284	83	1.3	
SD	87	60	7	0.3	
P value	0.072	0.579	0.255	0.939	

Achilles tendon approach, superficially to the superior flexor retinaculum and down to the Achilles tendon insertion. After proper pretensioning, FDL is attached to the calcaneus with a 5.0-mm metallic anchor and a no. 2 polyester polyethylene suture. The ideal positioning of the anchor is in the medial aspect of the posterior calcaneal tuberosity, approximately 2 cm inferior to its dorsal edge. To avoid impingement on the neurovascular bundle by the transferred tendon, the anchor should not be placed in the midline or lateral calcaneus. The FDL is tensioned to allow for 15° to 20° of ankle dorsiflexion, but the tendon is sutured with the ankle in 20° of plantarflexion.

In their retrospective review of 13 patients (15 feet), the investigators found significant changes in preoperative and postoperative visual analog scale (VAS), 36-Item Short Form Health Survey, and lower extremity functional scale scores. Furthermore, 12 patients (92%) could perform a single-leg heel rise test in the operated extremity, although there was a significant difference when comparing operated and uninvolved sides. One patient reported weakness for plantar flexion of the lesser toes, without balance or gait disturbances.[19]

Peroneus Brevis

First described in 1974,[20] the peroneus brevis tendon transfer also is a viable option for neglected Achilles tendon ruptures. The procedure is technically demanding but has proved useful. The technique, described by Maffulli and colleagues,[21] starts with a 10-cm to 12-cm skin incision made over the lateral border of the Achilles tendon. The sural nerve is identified and protected. The paratenon is incised in the midline and the stumps of the Achilles tendon are exposed. Scar tissue is excised to healthy tendon, and the gap is measured while maximally plantarflexing the ankle and pulling traction on the proximal tendon stump. Next, a small longitudinal incision is made in the lateral aspect of the floor of the Achilles tendon compartment to expose the distal portion of the peroneal muscle belly. The proximal peroneus brevis tendon is identified. A separate 2.5-mm longitudinal incision is made over the lateral base of the fifth metatarsal to identify the distal portion of the tendon. The tendon is detached from the base of the metatarsal and pulled through the proximal wound. The tendon then is passed through the distal stump of the Achilles tendon from lateral to medial and then passed through the proximal stump from medial to lateral. The repair then is sutured in place at each entry and exit point and reinforced with sutures between the musculotendinous junction of the peroneus brevis and the adjacent portion of the Achilles tendon. Interrupted sutures are used to approximate the ascending and descending limb of the peroneus brevis tendon.

Maffulli and colleagues[21] reported on their long-term outcomes of 16 patients who underwent peroneus brevis tendon for Achilles tendon defects up to 6.5 cm, with average follow-up of 15.5 years. No patients sustained a rerupture. The maximum calf circumference and isometric plantarflexion strength with the ankle in neutral were both significantly decreased, although patients did not perceive any weakness in strength in daily and leisurely activities. Complications reported included superficial infection, contralateral Achilles tendinopathy, hypersensitive surgical wounds, and hypertrophic scar.

In a case series by Miskulin and colleagues,[22] the investigators presented 5 patients who underwent peroneus brevis tendon transfer for chronic Achilles tendon ruptures. The average time to surgery from the initial injury was 19.8 weeks. They reported that the peak torque of plantar flexion increased in all patients (range, 21%–410%). Four patients were found to have an increase of the dorsal flexors peak torque (range, 31%–290%), whereas 1 patient showed a decrease (−37%). No patient experienced wound closure complications, postoperative pain, or functional limitations.

ALLOGRAFT

Multiple allografts have been described in the literature for neglected Achilles tendon ruptures, including peroneus brevis, hamstring, Achilles, and semitendinosus tendons.[23–26] Furthermore, Achilles tendon with a bone block also has been described,[27] which is the technique outlined in this article. In the technique described by So and colleagues,[27] a midline incision is made to the level of the paratenon. All of the diseased Achilles tendon then is sharply resected. After débridement, at least some portion of the native tendon should remain at the proximal graft attachment site to allow for adequate strength of suture repair. The posterior superior aspect of the calcaneus is resected in a distal-posterior to proximal-anterior direction under fluoroscopic guidance. The width can range from 1.2 cm to 2.5 cm at its insertion. After an initial resection is performed, the bone block can be placed on the posterior aspect of the calcaneus to gauge positioning of the allograft. At this time, the bone block allograft may be contoured to precisely match the contour of the resected calcaneus. After appropriate contouring of the bone block allograft, fixation using 4.5-mm and 5.5-mm cannulated screws are placed. Fluoroscopy is used to confirm appropriate alignment and placement of orthopedic hardware. The foot then is plantarflexed, and the proximal Achilles tendon is attached to the remaining proximal portion with an end-to-end repair. Before repair, the proximal musculotendinous stump is stimulated with electrocautery to confirm the presence of adequate muscle contraction. Repair is performed with nonabsorbable suture. Care must be taken to repair the allograft under physiologic tension. Excess allograft tendon is sharply removed.

In their case series of 2 patients, 1 patient with a follow-up of 8.5 years had a VAS score of 0, manual muscle strength of 5 out of 5, calf circumference equal to the nonoperative leg, and no gait disturbances. In their second case, with a follow-up of 9.7 years, the results were similar. The literature is sparse with respect to bone block Achilles allograft for treatment of chronic Achilles tendon ruptures so this technique should be reserved for those patients with large tendon gaps and when all other forms of repair have been exhausted.

SUMMARY

In conclusion, multiple reconstructive strategies exist for the treatment of neglected Achilles tendon ruptures. Choosing a treatment strategy typically depends on the quality of the existing tendon, size of the gap, and surgeon's comfort with each technique. In general, the treatment strategies achieve similar functional outcomes, as evidenced by the drastic improvement in functional outcome scores in almost every study. Regardless of the procedure chosen, patients should be counseled on the likelihood of generalized calf atrophy, deficits in ankle plantarflexion strength compared with the uninjured side, and the possibility of weakened hallux plantarflexion (eg, in patients who have undergone an FHL transfer). Patients still should expect to return to leisure and athletic activities, however, without functional deficits.

CLINICS CARE POINTS

- The normal size of an Achilles tendon is 4 mm to 6 mm; those tendons with chronic intrasubstance tendinopathy range anywhere from 7 mm to 16 mm from anteroposterior.
- Care must be taken to preserve the paratenon because the Achilles tendon has been shown to be quite avascular throughout its length despite being supplied from 3 different areas.

DISCLOSURES

Dr J.M. Cottom is a paid consultant for Arthrex.

SUPPLEMENTARY DATA

Supplementary data related to this article can be found online at https://doi.org/10.1016/j.cpm.2020.12.010.

REFERENCES

1. Egger AC, Berkowitz MJ. Achilles tendon injuries. Curr Rev Musculoskelet Med 2017;10(1):72–80.
2. Saini SS, Reb CW, Chapter M, et al. Achilles tendon disorders. J Am Osteopath Assoc 2015;115(11):670–6.
3. Kuwada GT. Classification of tendo Achillis rupture with consideration of surgical repair techniques. J Foot Surg 1990;29(4):361–5.
4. McQuilling JP, Sanders M, Poland L, et al. Dehydrated amnion/chorion improves achilles tendon repair in a diabetic animal model. Wounds 2019;31(1):19–25.
5. Arner O, Lindholm A. Subcutaneous rupture of the Achilles tendon; a study of 92 cases. Acta Chir Scand Suppl 1959;116(Supp 239):1–51.
6. Hsu AR, Jones CP, Cohen BE, et al. Clinical outcomes and complications of percutaneous achilles repair system versus open technique for acute achilles tendon ruptures. Foot Ankle Int 2015;36(11):1279–86.
7. McWilliam JR, Mackay G. The internal brace for midsubstance achilles ruptures. Foot Ankle Int 2016;37(7):794–800.
8. Cottom JM, Baker JS, Richardson PE, et al. Evaluation of a new knotless suture anchor repair in acute achilles tendon ruptures: a biomechanical comparison of three techniques. J Foot Ankle Surg 2017;56(3):423–7.
9. Abraham E, Pankovich AM. Neglected rupture of the Achilles tendon. Treatment by V-Y tendinous flap. J Bone Joint Surg Am 1975;57(2):253–5.
10. Elias I, Besser M, Nazarian LN, et al. Reconstruction for missed or neglected achilles tendon rupture with V-Y lengthening and flexor hallucis longus tendon transfer through one incision. Foot Ankle Int 2007;28(12):1238–48.
11. Christensen I. Rupture of the Achilles tendon; analysis of 57 cases. Acta Chir Scand 1953;106(1):50–60.
12. Peterson KS, Hentges MJ, Catanzariti AR, et al. Surgical considerations for the neglected or chronic achilles tendon rupture: a combined technique for reconstruction. J Foot Ankle Surg 2014;53(5):664–71.
13. Seker A, Kara A, Armagan R, et al. Reconstruction of neglected achilles tendon ruptures with gastrocnemius flaps: excellent results in long-term follow-up. Arch Orthop Trauma Surg 2016;136(10):1417–23.
14. Us AK, Bilgin SS, Aydin T, et al. Repair of neglected Achilles tendon ruptures: procedures and functional results. Arch Orthop Trauma Surg 1997;116(6–7):408–11.
15. Sanada T, Uchiyama E. Gravity equinus position to control the tendon length of reversed free tendon flap reconstruction for chronic achilles tendon rupture. J Foot Ankle Surg 2017;56(1):37–41.
16. Wapner KL, Pavlock GS, Hecht PJ, et al. Repair of chronic Achilles tendon rupture with flexor hallucis longus tendon transfer. Foot Ankle 1993;14(8):443–9.
17. Neufeld SK, Farber DC. Tendon transfers in the treatment of Achilles' tendon disorders. Foot Ankle Clin 2014;19(1):73–86.

18. Shinabarger AB, Manway JM, Nowak J, et al. Soft tissue fixation with a cortical button and interference screw: a novel technique in foot and ankle surgery. Foot Ankle Spec 2015;8(1):42–5.
19. de Cesar Netto C, Chinanuvathana A, Fonseca LF da, et al. Outcomes of flexor digitorum longus (FDL) tendon transfer in the treatment of Achilles tendon disorders. Foot Ankle Surg 2019;25(3):303–9.
20. Pérez Teuffer A. Traumatic rupture of the Achilles Tendon. Reconstruction by transplant and graft using the lateral peroneus brevis. Orthop Clin North Am 1974;5(1):89–93.
21. Maffulli N, Spiezia F, Pintore E, et al. Peroneus brevis tendon transfer for reconstruction of chronic tears of the Achilles tendon: a long-term follow-up study. J Bone Joint Surg Am 2012;94(10):901–5.
22. Miskulin M, Miskulin A, Klobucar H, et al. Neglected rupture of the Achilles tendon treated with peroneus brevis transfer: a functional assessment of 5 cases. J Foot Ankle Surg 2005;44(1):49–56.
23. Kocabey Y, Nyland J, Nawab A, et al. Reconstruction of neglected Achilles' tendon defect with peroneus brevis tendon allograft: a case report. J Foot Ankle Surg 2006;45(1):42–6.
24. Ellison P, Mason LW, Molloy A. Chronic Achilles tendon rupture reconstructed using hamstring tendon autograft. Foot (Edinb) 2016;26:41–4.
25. Cienfuegos A, Holgado MI, Díaz del Río JM, et al. Chronic Achilles rupture reconstructed with Achilles tendon allograft: a case report. J Foot Ankle Surg 2013; 52(1):95–8.
26. Sarzaeem MM, Lemraski MMB, Safdari F. Chronic Achilles tendon rupture reconstruction using a free semitendinosus tendon graft transfer. Knee Surg Sports Traumatol Arthrosc 2012;20(7):1386–91.
27. So E, Consul D, Holmes T. Achilles tendon reconstruction with bone block allograft:long-term follow-up of two cases. J Foot Ankle Surg 2019;58(4):779–84.

Os Trigonum Syndrome

Jeffrey E. McAlister, DPM[a],*, Usman Urooj, DPM, PGY-III[b]

KEYWORDS

- Os trigonum • Posterior ankle impingement syndrome • Steida process
- Flexor hallucis longus synovitis

KEY POINTS

- Os trigonum usually becomes symptomatic in active Individuals.
- Diagnosis of Os trigonum is made based on history, clinical exam and findings and imaging.
- Treatment may include conservative care. For more active population, surgical options maybe more suitable.

INTRODUCTION

In 1804, Rosenmuller first described the os trigonum as an accessory ossicle that failed to fuse to the posterolateral talar process.[1] Literature indicates that the prevalence of os trigonum syndrome ranges from 1.7% to 7%.[2] The talus bone has 2 posterior tubercles with a central groove.

Lateral tubercle of the posterior talus, or Stieda process, is larger in comparison to the medial tubercle. A secondary center of ossification of the lateral talar tubercle develops in the embryo during the second month of human gestation and becomes visible on radiographs at age 8 to 10 years in girls and 11 to 13 in boys. Secondary ossification center of this accessory ossicle typically fuse in the same year it becomes visible.

Os trigonum is a name given to an unfused secondary ossification center of the posterolateral talar tubercle. This failure of fusion of the secondary ossification center is reported to occur in 1.7% to 49% of the general population.[2,3] Os trigonum can also result from an acute fracture of the Stieda process also known as a Shepherd fracture. Os trigonum *syndrome* can also be referred to as *posterior ankle syndrome* and can be defined as an unfused secondary ossification center that becomes symptomatic from repetitive use or an injury. This syndrome can result from an overuse injury owing to repetitive plantar flexion stresses. Overuse or traumatic injury can lead to a fracture

[a] Phoenix Foot and Ankle Institute, 7301 East 2nd Street, Suite 206, Scottsdale, AZ 85251, USA;
[b] Department of Surgery-Podiatry, Carl T. Hayden Medical Center, 650 East Indian School Road, Phoenix, AZ 85012, USA
* Corresponding author.
E-mail address: Jeff.mcalister@gmail.com

Clin Podiatr Med Surg 38 (2021) 279–290
https://doi.org/10.1016/j.cpm.2020.12.011
0891-8422/21/© 2021 Elsevier Inc. All rights reserved.

podiatric.theclinics.com

of the Stieda process, cartilaginous synchondrosis disruption, or an avulsion injury of the posterior talofibular ligament. This posterior ankle impingement syndrome is most commonly seen in ballet dancers, swimmers, and soccer players because of repetitive pushoff maneuvers and hyper-plantarflexion injuries.

CLINICAL PRESENTATION AND PHYSICAL EXAMINATION

Routine history, when evaluating a patient, with posterior ankle syndrome should include sport-related activities and mechanism of injury. A thorough clinical examination involves both a weight-bearing and non-weight-bearing examination with highlights on gait analysis and reproduction of symptoms. Local edema should be assessed and neurovascular status integrity confirmed. Attention is directed at ankle stability, checking medial and lateral ankle static and dynamic stabilizers. Symptoms often may be referred to the Achilles or even mimic posterior tibial tendinitis. A Silfverskiold test may be performed to assess the range of motion of the posterior muscle group in the lower leg. Symptoms will also be deep and typically worsen with range of motion and weight-bearing. Tenderness should be confirmed along the posterior ankle, typically both medial and lateral, depending on severity. The symptomatic area can be ruled in with exquisite pain with hyper-plantarflexion or a heel thrush test. A heel thrush test elicits pain by "pinching" the talus between the posterior lip of the tibia and the superior aspect of the calcaneus. The flexor hallucis longus (FHL) tendon runs through the groove bordered medially and laterally by the 2 posterior talar tubercles. Therefore, tenderness with range of motion of the FHL tendon or with pushoff or propulsion may be noted. Tenderness with motion of the FHL tendon is indicative of tenosynovitis caused by rubbing alongside the injured posterior talus.

As previously mentioned, this syndrome is most commonly seen in ballet dancers, swimmers, and soccer players or in patients with jobs that require repetitive pushoff maneuvers. Although most commonly seen with sporting activities that involve repetitive plantar flexion maneuvers, the nonathletic population should not be ignored. In 2019, Kalbouneh and colleagues found that os trigonum syndrome should be suspected in nonathletic patients after an ankle sprain has been unresponsive to standard treatment. About 1.1% of acute ankle sprain patients developed an os trigonum syndrome. This finding can help identify the source of a patient's symptoms, leading to an accurate diagnosis, appropriate treatment, and reduction in the potential for chronic symptoms.[4] In 2018, D'Hooghe and colleagues[5] hypothesized that a lateral ligament ankle injury and thus instability would increase the likelihood for surgery in those athletes with os trigonum syndrome. Their study concluded that professional athletes with chronic lateral ankle ligament injury have 10 times greater risk of os trigonum syndrome compared with athletes with acute lateral ligament ankle injury.[6]

DIAGNOSIS AND DIFFERENTIAL DIAGNOSIS
Imaging

Radiographs and advanced imaging are recommended to rule in a synchondrosis or fracture of the posterior process of the talus as well as any soft tissue irritation (**Fig. 1**). An os trigonum is plainly seen radiographically on a lateral view and can be seen between the posterior malleolus and superior calcaneus in full plantarflexion. Advanced imaging is then ordered to confirm diagnosis and assess any FHL tenosynovitis. MRI can also be used to identify any abnormal manifestations, such as bone marrow edema, a fracture line, or fluid in the posterior lateral talar tubercle.

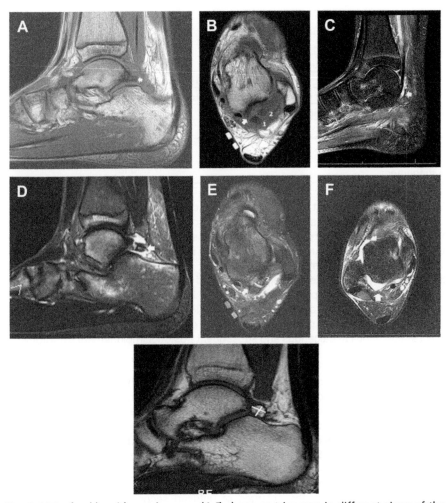

Fig. 1. MRI of ankle with os trigonum. (*A-F*) shows os trigonum in different views of the MRI. X represents os trigonum. (*From* Rungprai C, Tennant JN, Phisitkul P. Disorders of the Flexor Hallucis Longus and Os Trigonum. Clin Sports Med. 2015;34(4):741-759. https://doi. org/10.1016/j.csm.2015.06.005; with permission.)

It can also assist in evaluating any associated FHL and or ankle pathologic condition. *Computed tomography is useful when trying to assess for fracture lines in the picture of a talar fracture. Bone scans and PET scans are typically not useful in this diagnosis.*

When a patient presents to the clinic with posterior ankle pain, a list of differentials should be considered. As summarized in **Table 1**, some of these include soft tissue impingement, such as scar tissue resulting from sprains, muscle impingement (accessory muscles, such as peroneus quadrates and accessory flexor digitorum longus), Shepherd fracture, Achilles tendinitis, FHL tendinitis or tenosynovitis, retrocalcaneal bursitis, osteochondritis dissecans, osteoarthritis, subtalar coalition, stress fracture, Sever's disease, bone tumor, such as osteoid osteoma, or nerve entrapment, such as tarsal tunnel or sural nerve entrapment syndrome[7] (see **Table 1**).

Table 1		
Differential diagnoses for posterior ankle pain		
Posterior Ankle Impingement	**Acute Trauma**	**Other Posterior Ankle Pathologic Conditions**
Scar tissue impingement	Shepherd fracture	Achilles tendinitis
Accessory ligament impingement	Synchondrosis disruption	FHL tendinitis/tenosynovitis
Accessory muscle impingement	FHL rupture	Sever's disease
Osteochondral lesion		Osteoid osteoma

Management

Conservative

Treatment or management of os trigonum can be classified into conservative and surgical care. Conservative treatment may include avoidance of aggravating activity, RICE protocol, anti-inflammatory medications, corticosteroid injections, and physical therapy. Albisetti and colleagues[8] demonstrated the benefits of rest, avoidance of aggravating factors, anti-inflammatory medications, and physical therapy. The study consisted of a physical therapy regimen focused on strengthening and stretching the deep lower leg muscles (posterior tibial tendon, FHL tendon, flexor digitorum longus tendon, and peroneal tendons). The goal of this study was to minimize the use of big posterior leg muscles during plantar flexor motions of the ankle, thereby decreasing the direct action of pull at calcaneus and subsequent posterior impingement symptoms.

Surgical

This treatment may be considered after failure of 3 to 6 months of conservative treatment or in an athlete or dancer who wants to get back to activity faster.

Os trigonum is a structural problem; goal of the conservative treatment is to get control of inflammation, which should result in improvement in symptoms. If there is no improvement in symptoms with conservative treatment, surgical options may be considered. Surgical options may be the necessary route for the active population such as athlete or dances who wishes to continue training. Surgical intervention, in many cases, is simple in regards to what needs to be done, that is, excision of the offending agent, which is the enlarged or unfused secondary ossification center. Essentially there are 3 ways of excision: posterior endoscopy, arthroscopy or open procedure.

Endoscopic approach

The endoscopic approach was first described by Powell and colleagues in 2000.[9] Morelli and colleagues[6] in 2017 showed excellent results with endoscopic excision of os trigonum. The purpose of this retrospective study was to present the clinical results of excision of symptomatic os trigonum using an endoscopic procedure in professional ballet dancers. They had a total of 12 professional dancers who had a pure os trigonum–related posterior ankle pain with unsatisfactory improvement after a rehabilitative protocol lasting greater than 6 months. A 4.5-mm arthroscope was used with standard posterolateral and posteromedial arthroscopic hindfoot portals on either side of the Achilles tendon, at the level of the fibular tip. Then, a C-arm was used to locate the os trigonum. After localization of the os trigonum, it was debrided by tethering the soft tissue and then was integrally removed. A final inspection and dynamic visualization, using the C-arm, were completed to confirm the excision of the ossicle. Two weeks postoperatively, patients were allowed to weight-bear and to increase their physical activity. At 4 weeks, they were allowed to return to running, and at 6 weeks, training for dance was allowed. At the final follow-up examination, none of the patients were experiencing pain with plantarflexion and were able to return to full dance activity with good success. The results of their study are listed in **Table 2**. They were able to show that postoperatively no patient showed signs of local tenderness or swelling, and the forced plantarflexion findings were negative for any discomfort. The Tegner score, American Orthopedic Foot and Ankle Society (AOFAS) score, and visual analog scale (VAS) score were all statistically significant.

Ling and Walsh in 2020 also showed excellent results with a 2-portal endoscopic technique for posterior ankle pain surgical management. They also used the 2-portal system. They used a 4.5-mm shaver to remove soft tissue. Then, the fragment was able to be mobilized in most cases; if not, then a small osteotome was introduced through the medial portal to mobilize the fragment. The FHL tendon was debrided if synovitis was noted. The aim of their study was to evaluate the short-, medium-, and long-term outcomes with this technique. This retrospective case series analysis included a mean follow-up time of 4.8 years. Of the 52 patients, 49 (94%) were able to return to their previous sport or physical activity, with the mean time taken to return to training being 5.8 months. The mean work and sporting function scores improved from preoperatively 5.9 to postoperatively 9.6 points and preoperatively 2.9 to postoperatively 8.8 points, respectively. There were no postoperative infections or any other major complications. This study provided strong evidence supporting the use of hindfoot endoscopy in the treatment of posterior ankle impingement syndrome in athletes.[10]

Arthroscopic approach (subtalar arthroscopy)

This approach was first introduced by Marumoto and Ferkel,[11] who reported on an arthroscopic excision in 1997 that led to shorter recovery times than compared with the open approach. A 2.7-mm arthroscope is used for inspection of the subtalar joint through the anterolateral and posterolateral portals, followed by excision of the ossicle. This approach is more challenging because of the small working space at the subtalar joint. This technique is useful when other anterior ankle pathologic conditions are also present.[11–13]

A study in 2013 by Park and colleagues involved 23 patients who were treated with arthroscopic resection of the os trigonum. Patients in this study were soccer, basketball, baseball players, or gymnasts. Os trigonum syndrome in all of these patients was due to traumatic ankle injury. The mean follow-up was 18 months. Postoperatively, the AOFAS score increased from 71.3 to 94.7; the mean VAS pain score went from 6.7 to 1.5, and average plantar flexion increased from 28.8° to 42.5°. Average return to sports was 6.7 weeks. No major complications were reported for these patients.

In a study in 2015,[14] Weiss and colleagues also showed favorable arthroscopic excision of os trigonum. Their procedure involved ankle and subtalar joint arthroscopy. Out of 24 patients, 21 had isolated os trigonum excisions. Mean follow-up was 26 months. Average AOFAS score changed significantly from 55.3 preoperatively to 92.3 postoperatively. Patients reported full activity at an average of 1.5 months with no limitations at an average of 7.8 months after surgery. The only complication that was noted was one case of posterior tibial nerve calcaneal branch neuropraxia.

Endoscopic versus arthroscopic approach

Ahn and colleagues[2] did a comparison of the anterior versus posterior excision in 2013. They compared the outcomes in 28 patients treated with either the arthroscopic anterior approach or the posterior endoscopic approach. Both groups had substantially improved VAS and AOFAS scores postoperatively, with no significant difference

Table 2
Outcomes of surgical management of posterior ankle impingement from recent literature

Study, Year	No. of Patients	Average Age (y)	Technique	Mean F/U (mo/y)	Outcomes
Ahn et al,[2] 2013	Arthroscopic: 16, and endoscopic: 12	10 for both groups	Arthroscopic and endoscopic	Arthroscopic: 29, and endoscopic: 30	Arthroscopic: • VAS: preoperative: 6.3 to postoperative: 1.2 • AOFAS: preoperative: 64 to postoperative: 89 • Return to sports: 7.5 wk Endoscopic: • VAS: preoperative: 6.7 to postoperative: 1.2 • AOFAS: preoperative: 64.8 to postoperative: 89.9 • Return to sports: 8.0
Park et al,[7] 2013	23	25	Arthroscope	18	AOFAS: Preoperative: 71.3 to postoperative: 94.7 VAS: preoperative: 6.7 to postoperative: 1.5 Return to sports: 6.7 wk
Weiss et al,[19] 2015	24	36	Arthroscope	26	• AOFAS: preoperative: 55.3 to postoperative: 92.3 • AOFAS function: preoperative: 17.1 to postoperative: 33.8
Ballal et al,[20] 2016	35	Endoscopic: 18 Open: 20	Endoscope and open	12	Endoscopic: Return to full dance: 9.8 wk Open: Return to full dance: 14.9 wk
Morelli et al,[6] 2017	12	27	Endoscope	39 ± 20.6	AOFAS: 68–96[a] VAS: 8–2.5[a]

Study					

Georgiannos and Bisbinas,[21] 2017	52	26	Open (group A) vs endoscope (group B)	60	Group A:
					  AOFAS: 66–87 (5 y)
					  VAS: 43–92 (5 y)
					  Mean return to sports: 9 wk
					Group B:
					  AOFAS: 65–93 (5 y)
					  VAS: 45–93 (5 y)
					  Mean return to sports: 4 wk

Ling and Walsh,[22] 2020	52	21	Endoscope	60 (~5 y)	Pain score: 7.5–0.9 • Function at work score: 5.9–9.1 • Sporting function score: 2.9–8.0 • SFRFFI: 84–6.7

Abbreviation: SFRFFI, short form of the revised foot function index.
[a] Statistically significant.
Data from Refs.[2,6,7,19–22]

between the groups. In addition, the mean surgical time for arthroscopy was 39.4 minutes and for endoscopy it was 34.8 minutes. Return to sport was similar for both groups. The investigators concluded that both techniques are safe and effective but also stated that arthroscopy (anterior approach) is more demanding, especially in cases of a large os trigonum, with a failure rate of 12.5%. They recommended the use of arthroscope when other pathologic conditions of the ankle are also present.

Open os trigonum excision

Posterolateral approach. A 4- to 5-cm straight incision is made posterior to the lateral malleolus and medial to the peroneal tendons. Then, after careful soft tissue dissection, the sural nerve is identified and retracted. Next, the posterior capsule of the ankle joint is identified and incised. At this time, the os trigonum is identified and removed using a rongeur, an osteotome, or a saw. The rasp is used to smooth the remaining bone, with bone wax application to control bleeding. Irrigation is performed next, and closure is performed.

Posteromedial approach. With the limb in external rotation, an incision approximately 1 cm anterior to the medial aspect of the Achilles tendon is made. With this technique, extreme care must be taken to protect the neurovascular bundle. Next, blunt dissection is directed anterolaterally toward the FHL. The FHL sheath is identified and released. The os trigonum is identified and removed using a rongeur, an osteotome, or a saw. A rasp can be used to smooth the remaining bone.

Heyer and colleagues[15] in 2017 described their steps of the posteromedial approach as starting with a 3-cm slightly curvilinear longitudinal incision made midway between the posterior aspect of the medial malleolus and the anterior aspect of the Achilles tendon. Then, the FHL tendon is palpated, and the flexor retinaculum is exposed and incised. The neurovascular bundle is retracted anteriorly, exposing the FHL tendon and sheath. Next, FHL tenolysis or tenosynovectomy is performed, if needed. Then, the FHL is retracted anteriorly; a capsulotomy is performed over the os trigonum, and the os trigonum is excised. Last, the capsule is repaired, and closure is performed.[16]

Endoscopic versus open

Ballal and colleagues in 2016 showed the benefits of endoscopy over open procedures in professional ballet dancers. In their study, they concluded that although both techniques are safe and effective in the treatment of symptomatic os trigonum, in professional ballet dancers, endoscopic excision of os trigonum offers a quicker time to full return to activity. Their results are shown in **Table 1**.[3]

Georgiannos and Bisbinas in 2017 concluded that both open procedure and endoscopic approach yield good outcomes, but complication rates are lower with endoscopic treatment, and the time to return to full activities is shorter. Their results are shown in **Table 1**.[17]

POSTOPERATIVE REHABILITATION

Postoperative care may be different from surgeon to surgeon and depends on the extent of work that was done. In general, a compression bandage is applied after surgical intervention, and usually patients are allowed to weight-bear to avoid any scar tissue build up, which can potentially delay patient's return to activity.

COMPLICATIONS OF SURGICAL INTERVENTION

Complications from the surgical approach in os trigonum excision may lead to injury of the sural nerve, reported at a rate of 3.4% to 8.3%, with the arthroscopic approach,

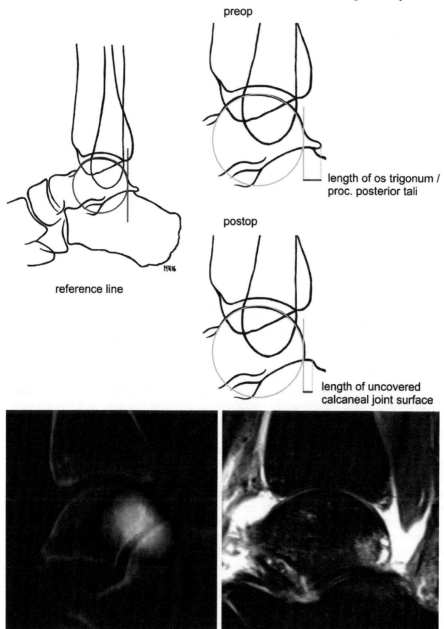

Fig. 2. An ankle showing impact on subtalar joint post os trigonum resection. The red line indicates location of os trigonum. Red circle indicates subtalar joint and or Talus. Postop, postoperative; preop, preoperative; proc, procedure. (*From* Frigg A, Maquieira G, Horisberger M. Painful stress reaction in the posterior subtalar joint after resection of os trigonum or posterior talar process. *Int Orthop.* 2017;41(8):1585-1592. https://doi.org/10.1007/s00264-017-3489-z; with permission.)

versus 6.3% to 19.5% with the open approach. With the posteromedial approach, there is a risk of injury to the neurovascular bundle. Tibial nerve injury can also occur and was reported at a rate of 6.7% in the open approach versus 11.1% in the arthroscopic approach. Wound infections can also result with superficial wound infection reported in 3.3% to 6.7% of the wounds and deep wound infection in 3.3% of the wounds with the arthroscopic approach versus only superficial wound infection reported in 2.4% of the wounds in the open surgical approach.[18] Damage to the joint surfaces can also occur or posterior subtalar joint stress reaction. In a 2017 study, Frigg and colleagues showed that the surgical resection of os trigonum or posterior talar process had a complication rate of 13% with painful stress reactions in the posterior subtalar joint during follow-up, which can be career ending in some athletes. In this study, they identified that after os trigonum excision, the talar radius ends inside the subtalar joint (**Fig. 2**). In such cases, the resection should be made sparingly, preferably not anterior into the subtalar joint, and patients must be informed about possible future complications.

SUMMARY

Os trigonum is the result of an unfused secondary ossification center or a fracture of an elongated lateral talar tubercle. It can become symptomatic following overuse, following ankle trauma, or in athletes and dancers performing repetitive forced plantar flexion at the ankle joint. Patient may present to the clinic with pain to the posterior ankle, which will exacerbate with plantarflexion. Pain with range of motion of the FHL tendon may also be a presenting symptom. Diagnosis should be based on presenting history, physical examination, and imaging. Conservative treatment includes RICE protocol, anti-inflammatory medications, physical therapy, and steroid injections. If conservative care is not improving the patient's symptoms, surgical intervention may be considered.

Three techniques are available for surgical intervention: arthroscopic or endoscopic techniques and open surgical excision. Overall, the 3 techniques improve function and provide a high rate of return to sport. Recent literature indicates that, although more demanding, arthroscopic or endoscopic techniques report a quicker return to sport or patient activity in comparison to open procedure. Some advantages of open and endoscopic techniques include the ability to manage larger ossicles, less demanding, and reduced to no damage to the joint surfaces. With the arthroscopic technique, additional posterior ankle pathologic conditions can be addressed during the same operating time, but with this technique, damage to the subtalar joint surfaces can lead to other ankle pathologic condition, such as subtalar joint arthritis. When comparing endoscopic and arthroscopic techniques, associated complications rates are similar and typically include injury to the sural and tibial nerves and infection. Results of some of the recent studies with these techniques are shown in **Table 2**.

Os trigonum is a structural problem of the posterior talus. Conservative measures can be taken, but if the patient is active or is involved in activities like dancing, sports, or any activity that requires repetitive plantarflexion, surgical intervention is recommended. Literature indicates that approximately 40% of the patients eventually require surgical intervention because of intractable hindfoot pain. Open excision of the os trigonum can be used, but recent literature indicates endoscopic technique leads to faster recovery, faster return to activity, and fewer complications. A recent systematic review by Smyt and colleagues[23] showed the advantages of the endoscopic approach over the open approach, including lower complication rates, less blood loss, shorter recovery time, less postoperative pain, and comparable functional outcomes. Arthroscopic technique may also be used, but this technique comes with a relatively steep learning curve.

CLINICS CARE POINTS

- Os trigonum syndrome diagnosis is typically a diagnosis of exclusion, and advanced imaging is useful in ruling in the pathologic condition.
- Arthroscopic approaches have significantly less complications and faster return to sport.
- Flexor hallucis longus pathologic condition should be recognized early in the treatment pathway.

PEARLS AND PITFALLS

- Os trigonum, when enlarged or with repetitive injury from use, can become symptomatic. Patients' history combined with physical examination is of the utmost importance to develop a correct diagnosis.
- Clinical findings and proper imaging can help in either confirming or ruling out symptomatic os trigonum or any associated pathologic condition.
- Surgical treatment is probably the most suitable for symptomatic os trigonum.
- The endoscopic approach versus open approach has its pros and cons. The endoscopic approach allows for less trauma to the surrounding tissues and possible damage to the neurovascular or surrounding structures.

REFERENCES

1. Marotta JJ, Micheli LJ. Os trigonum impingement in dancers. Am J Sports Med 1992;20:533–6.
2. Ahn JH, Kim Y-C, Kim H-Y. Arthroscopic versus posterior endoscopic excision of a symptomatic os trigonum. Am J Sports Med 2013;41(5):1082–9.
3. Lopez Valerio V, Seijas R, Alvarez P, et al. Endoscopic repair of posterior ankle impingement syndrome due to os trigonum in soccer players. Foot Ankle Int 2015;36(1):70–4.
4. Kushare I, Kastan K, Allhabadi S. Posterior ankle impingement-an underdiagnosed cause of ankle pain in pediatric patients. World J Orthop 2019;10:364–70.
5. D'Hooghe P, Alkhelaifi K, Almusa E, et al. Chronic lateral ankle instability increases the likelihood for surgery in athletes with os trigonum syndrome. Knee Surg Sports Traumatol Arthrosc 2019;27:2814–7.
6. Morelli F, Mazza D, Serlorenzi P, et al. Endoscopic excision of symptomatic os trigonum in professional dancers. J Foot Ankle Surg 2017;56:22–5.
7. Park CH, Kim SY, Kim JR, et al. Arthroscopic excision of a symptomatic os trigonum in a lateral decubitus position. Foot Ankle Int 2013;34(7):990–4.
8. Albisetti W, Ometti M, Pascale V, et al. Clinical evaluation and treatment of posterior impingement in dancers. Am J Phys Med Rehabil 2009;349–54.
9. Powell BD, Minton T, Cooper. Ankle MRI and arthroscopy correlation with cartilaginous defects and symptomatic os trigonum. Sports Med Arthrosc Rev 2017;25(4):237–45.

10. Kalbouneh HM, Omar AL, Alsalem M, et al. Incidence of symptomatic os trigonum among nonathletic patients with ankle sprain. Surg Radiol Anat 2019;41: 1433–9.

11. Marumoto JM, Ferkel RD. Arthroscopic excision of the os trigonum: a new technique with preliminary clinical results. Foot Ankle Int 1997;18:777–84.

12. Galla M, Lobenhoffer P. Technique and results of arthroscopic treatment of posterior ankle impingement. Foot Ankle Surg 2011;17:79–84.

13. Corte-Real NM, Moreira RM, Guerra-Pinto F. Arthroscopic treatment of tenosynovitis of the flexor hallucis longus tendon. Foot Ankle Int 2012;33:1108–12.

14. Rungparai C, Tennant JN, Phisitkul P. Disorders of the flexor hallucis longus and os trigonum. Clin Sports Med 2015;34:741–59.

15. Heyer JH, Dai AZ, Rose DJ. Excision of os trigonum in dancers via an open posteromedial approach. Foot Ankle Int 2017;38:27–35.

16. Frigg A, Maquieira G, Horisberger M. Painful stress reaction in the posterior subtalar joint after resection of os trigonum or posterior talar process. Int Orthop 2017;41:1585–92.

17. Grambar ST. Imaging of common arthroscopic pathology of the ankle. Clin Podiatr Med Surg 2016;33:493–502.

18. Nault M-L, Kocher MS, Micheli LJ. Os trigonum syndrome. J Am Acad Orthrop Surg 2014;22:545–53.

19. Weiss WM, Sanders EJ, crates JM, et al. Arthroscopic excision of a symptomatic os trigonum. J Arthrosc Relat Surg 2015;31:11.

20. Ballal MS, Roche A, Brodrick A, et al. Posterior endoscopic excision of os trigonum in professional national ballet dancers. J Foot Ankle Surg 2016;55:927–30.

21. Georgiannos D, Bisbinas I. Endoscopic versus open excision of os trigonum for the treatment of posterior ankle impingement syndrome in an athletic population. Am J Sports Med 2017;45(6):1388–94.

22. Ling CT, Walsh SJ. Outcomes of a 2-portal endoscopic technique for osseous lesions resulting in posterior ankle impingement syndrome. J Foot Ankle Surg 2020; 59(5):938–41.

23. Smyt NA, Zwiers R, Wiegerinck JI, et al. Posterior hindfoot arthroscopy: a review. American journal of Sports Medicine 2014;225–34.

Moving?

Make sure your subscription moves with you!

To notify us of your new address, find your **Clinics Account Number** (located on your mailing label above your name), and contact customer service at:

Email: journalscustomerservice-usa@elsevier.com

800-654-2452 (subscribers in the U.S. & Canada)
314-447-8871 (subscribers outside of the U.S. & Canada)

Fax number: 314-447-8029

Elsevier Health Sciences Division
Subscription Customer Service
3251 Riverport Lane
Maryland Heights, MO 63043

*To ensure uninterrupted delivery of your subscription, please notify us at least 4 weeks in advance of move.

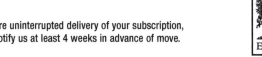

Printed and bound by CPI Group (UK) Ltd, Croydon, CR0 4YY

03/10/2024

01040481-0013